Thorsons
calorie
counter

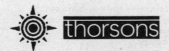

Thorsons
An Imprint of HarperCollins*Publishers*
77–85 Fulham Palace Road
Hammersmith, London W6 8JB

The website address is:
www.thorsonselement.com

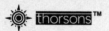 thorsons™

and *Thorsons* are trademarks of
HarperCollins*Publishers* Limited

Published by Thorsons 1995
This edition 2003

10 9 8 7 6 5 4 3

© Virtual City Associates 1995

A catalogue record for this book
is available from the British Library

ISBN 0 00 714746 5

Printed and bound in Great Britain by
Clays Ltd, St Ives plc, Bungay

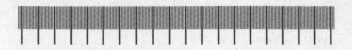

Contents

Acknowledgements v
How to use this book vi
Introduction vii

Bread 1
Cakes and Biscuits 12
Cereals 24
Crisps and Snacks 30
Dairy Products 34
Desserts 51
Drinks:
   Alcoholic 61
   Hot 62
   Non-alcoholic 63
Ethnic Foods 83
Fast Foods 89
Fats and Oils 104
Fish 107
Fruit 116
Ice-cream 125
Jams, Spreads, Sauces and Pickles 132
Meat and Poultry 140
Nuts 150

Processed Meats: Sausages, Salamis and Pâtés   155
Ready-made Meals   160
Rice, Pasta and Pizza   170
Sandwiches   182
Soups   188
Sugar, Syrups, Confectionery and Cereal Bars   195
Vegetables, Pulses and Prepared Salads   205
Vegetarian Dishes   219

Medical Warning

This book is for the basically healthy adult who wishes to lose (or gain) modest amounts of weight. Every calorie-controlled diet should also contain a well-balanced range of essential nutrients. People who have, or have relatives with, diabetes, high blood-pressure, heart disease or allergies of any kind, or who have suffered from any other serious disease, should seek medical advice before trying any form of dieting. There are also a number of illnesses that can result in weight gain or weight loss, which a diet alone will not address. Children, pregnant women and those in athletic programmes should also only diet on medical advice. The text in this book should be read in its entirety. In fact, if you have the slightest doubt, consult a doctor or qualified nutritionist.

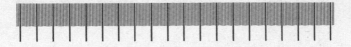

Acknowledgements

The nutritional material in this book has come from a variety of manufacturers, supermarkets, on-line information databases, and UK and US official sources. All brand names are hereby acknowledged. Particular help was received from Allied Bakeries Limited, Asda Stores Ltd, Baxters of Speyside Limited, Birds Eye Wall's Limited, Boots The Chemists Ltd, Brooke Bond Foods Ltd, Budgens Stores Limited, C Shippam Limited, Cadbury Ltd, Campbell Grocery Products Limited, Co-op Wholesale Society, Dairy Crest Limited, H J Heinz Company Ltd, Holland and Barrett, J A Sharwood & Co Ltd, John West Foods Limited, Kellogg Company of Great Britain Ltd, Kraft General Foods Ltd, Marks and Spencer plc, Nestlé UK Ltd, Northumbrian Fine Foods plc, Reckitt & Colman Products Limited, Safeway Stores plc, Sainsbury's plc, Sovereign Chicken Limited, St Ivel, The Jacob's Bakery Limited, The New Covent Garden Soup Co Ltd, UB (Ross Young's) Ltd, United Biscuits (UK) Limited, W Jordan (Cereals) Ltd, Waitrose Limited, and Whole Earth Foods Ltd. The UK official source was McCance and Widdowson: *The Composition of Foods* (Fifth Edition), used by permission of the Royal Society of Chemistry and the Comptroller of Her Majesty's Stationery Office. We'd like to acknowledge the editorial assistance of Sam Edwards.

How to Use This Book

- Read the primer on calorie counting, diet and nutrition beginning on page ix.
- Weigh yourself and compare your weight with the figures in the tables beginning on page xix.
- Take a look at your lifestyle and eating patterns, using the information on pages xxi–xxvi, and calculate the amount of energy you use up during your average day from the figures in the tables beginning on page xxii.
- Analyse your existing diet and estimate your daily energy intake from the foods you eat from the figures in the tables beginning on page 2.
- Set a realistic target for weight loss (or weight gain).
- Design or adapt a diet that will meet that target, using your analysis of your lifestyle and eating patterns and the calorie values in the schemes beginning on page xxix.

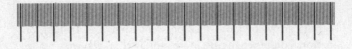

Introduction

Calorie Counting

According to a Gallup opinion poll, at least 20 per cent of the UK population is at any one time trying to slim; 59 per cent of men and 60 per cent of women think they are overweight.

The idea of calorie counting flows in and out of fashion. Any number of diet books offer allegedly simple rules for weight control: lists of 'good' and 'bad' foods, collections of recipes, miracle ingredients, and so on. But if they work at all, at the back of all of them someone somewhere is counting calories.

The drawback of so many of these schemes is their lack of flexibility; the advantage of a guide to calories is that you possess the basic information from which to adapt an existing plan or formulate your own.

Flexibility is more important now than ever because the life-styles most of us lead today are very different from those described in most diet books. They nearly all make an assumption: that our eating habits are centred on 'three square meals a day'. Implicitly all the advice given concentrates on changing the foods we eat during those three meals to reduce their calorific content. The fact is, many of us don't eat in that way at all – we 'snack' and we 'munch', that is, we are abandoning many formal meals and simply eat when we feel hungry.

Sales of chilled foods, the basis of so much convenience eating, grows by almost 12 per cent each year. In fact, our national diet is changing more rapidly than you may realize. All of us are buying less basic or generic food in favour of convenience products. Compared with 10 years ago we are buying 16 per cent less unprocessed meat. Sales of fresh and frozen fish fell in favour of cooked varieties. We are also buying fewer fresh vegetables, other than those that can be eaten immediately, a fall of over 20 per cent during the aforementioned decade. Only three per cent of us were vegetarians in 1986; that had doubled to 6 per cent by 1991 and now over 10 per cent of the population have abandoned meat.

Any diet plan which ignores these important social changes is probably not going to work.

Our changed lifestyles mean that both sides of the 'calorie-controlled diet' equation – our energy needs as a result of *how we spend our day* and our energy intake in the form of *what we eat* – have undergone profound alterations. Here, in a pocketable form, you'll be able to make your plans – and continue to live with them.

> Although people who diet normally wish to reduce their weight, some people need to gain weight – this book is for you as well.

Our Changing Lifestyles

Let's look at the social changes that were mentioned a little more closely; you may be able to recognize yourself in them. Many people still think that the 'normal' living arrangement consists of a family made up of a male adult, a female adult and one to two children. In fact, only one quarter of all UK households fall into this pattern. There are actually more households made up of just one person. Another 27 per cent are married couples with no children.

Now, if you live by yourself, conventional meals can sometimes be a bit of a bother – you may skip some in exchange for several snacks or take-aways. If you have no children you may feel less pressure always to eat at the same time, or mostly at the same place.

Work patterns also dictate our eating habits. Women make up nearly half of the work-force. We know the reasons well enough: a mixture of greater emancipation and a desire for a proper career – and an economic need to support the family. But a working woman approaches meals and meal preparation very differently from one whose main role is to look after the house and family. Again: many of us, men and women, are expected by our employers to work shifts. Nearly half of those employed work at weekends, 12 per cent do shift work based on the ordinary working day, and just under 2 per cent work nights. All of this has an enormous effect on *when* we eat as well as *what* we eat. This affects not only those who actually do the shift work, but everyone who lives with them, including children. Working in shifts means eating in shifts. There is a hidden hazard here, for slimmers: you may tend to eat with your loved ones as well as when you yourself are hungry – simply as a way of sharing some time with them.

There has been one other change during the last decade: many of us are having to travel longer distances to work. Some of us have voluntarily abandoned the inner suburbs in order to live in a healthier and cleaner environment; others have found that a house or flat big enough for their needs is just too expensive in the city. Longer commutes means abandoned breakfasts, sneaked snacks in the morning, later evening meals and, to compensate, more sneaked snacks in the late afternoon. The energy content of many favourite snacks can cause severe disruption to any diet plan.

This changed lifestyle also affects our patterns of hunger and appetite – we may feel hungry at times of the day when it is inconvenient to prepare and eat 'healthy' food. Our stomachs crave satisfaction when all that is available is instant junk food. Unless we are very aware of what is going on, any controlled diet scheme will soon fall to pieces. What is worse, many of us are sufficiently weak-willed to tell ourselves that such snacks don't really count: 'It doesn't matter that I had a quick packet of crisps or a biscuit, because my main meal of the day came with a "Low Calorie" label on it.' Check out the calorie tables for crisps and biscuits in this book, and see if you can still kid yourself!

The food industry – both manufacturers and retailers – have risen to the challenge of our new lifestyles. Chill-cooked (or half-cooked) foods, new packaging methods, and new semi-instant foods to be cooked rapidly in microwaves have all become occasional parts (and sometimes staples) of our diet. The food and supermarket industries refer to these as 'recipe dishes', but the term 'ready-made meals' has been used in this book.

The traditional formal meal hasn't completely disappeared of course, and it still plays an important role in all our lives – but look carefully at the last week or two of your life: how much of your diet was made up of informal snacking and munching?

Calorie Counting: A Quick Primer

This is not meant to be a full-blown guide to nutrition, but some explanations are essential if this book is to help you.

A calorie is a measure of the energy content of food. All foods have a calorific value and contribute to keeping the body going. A high calorific value means that there is a lot of energy locked up in the food which the body can convert. The various demands we make of our bodies – breathing, walking, talking, running, lifting and so on – all require energy, and this too can be measured in calories.

(Strictly speaking, the scientific unit of the energy is the Joule. If you look at the nutritional tables on most food packages you will find that energy values are expressed both in calories and in Joules. One calorie is the amount of heat required to raise the temperature of 1 gram of water by 1 degree centigrade. Since that is a very small amount of heat, the convenient unit for nutritional calculations is actually the kilocalorie, 1000 calories, abbreviated to kcal. So what we call calories are in fact kilocalories. The Joule is also too small for convenient use and nutritionists operate in kiloJoule units (kJ). The conversion factor is: 1 kilocalorie equals 4.184kJ.)

The principles of the calorie-controlled diet are perfectly simple: using the set of tables beginning on page xxiii you first take a look at your daily activities and calculate your individual energy requirements. Using the main Calorie Counter tables (beginning on page 2) you identify the energy content of the food you eat. In ideal circumstances the two figures should be identical. If you take in more food energy than your body burns up, some of it will be evacuated when you use the toilet, but some will stay in your body, typically deposited as fat, and your weight will increase. If you don't eat enough of the right sort of energy-giving food, then your body will have to draw on its own resources and use up existing stores of fat. Essentially, that's what you make your body do when you go on a traditional slimming diet.

Like many simple explanations, some important details are overlooked here, however.

First, there is of course more to food than its energy content. We require substantial amounts of water, both as a liquid, and 'trapped' or integrated into solid foods. Besides water, we require a wide range of vitamins and minerals. We also need a collection of proteins, and although proteins are one of the main sources of energy, quite apart from this they are essential to life. We must also have fibre (strictly speaking, fibre isn't a food because it is not ingested, however the alimentary canal requires it in order to function properly and ingest the 'true' foods).

So: you can't base a diet solely on calorie counting. Indeed, one of the many dangers of crash weight-loss courses is that the body ends up lacking essential nutrients. Whatever your plans, you must have what nutritionists call a 'well-balanced diet'. In general terms, this means eating a broad range of fresh foods, with an emphasis on uncooked (or only slightly cooked) fruit and vegetables. These foods should bring you all the proteins, vitamins and minerals your body needs.

Second, the way in which the body actually handles food is rather more complicated than the simple 'energy in /energy out' explanation.

The energy-supplying ingredients in food are: proteins, carbohydrates, fats and alcohol. Alcohol isn't normally thought of as a food because of its other, well-known effects, but it does supply energy.

Protein

Protein is made up of amino acids. There are 20 key amino acids. Eight of these are called essential amino acids because their nutrients cannot be manufactured by the body and must come from the outside, from our diet. Excess protein taken in is burned for energy. One gram of protein burned for its energy contains four calories.

Carbohydrate

Carbohydrates are the body's main source of energy. Other energy nutrients must be converted to carbohydrate before the body can use them. Carbohydrates provide glucose ready for the body to burn. But the body can also convert fat and protein to glucose, and will do so if the need arises. This is why starvation causes muscle tissue to waste away: living muscle proteins are burned for their energy. This takes place after the main fat stores in the body have been exhausted.

Carbohydrates can be classed as simple or complex. A simple carbohydrate is a mono- or di-saccharide. Examples of simple carbohydrates are glucose, fructose (found in fruit), sucrose and lactose (found in milk). Complex carbohydrates are polysaccharides, long chains of glucose molecules, more commonly referred to as starch. These take much longer to digest, because the body has to take them apart, one molecule at a time. One gram of carbohydrate contains four calories of energy, and people require a minimum of about 100 grams a day.

Fats

Fats are a concentrated energy source, yielding nine calories per gram, compared to the four per gram found in protein and carbohydrate. Nutritionally, fats exist in three different chemical states: saturated, monounsaturated and polyunsaturated. Generally, the more unsaturated a given fatty acid, the more liquid the fat is. Saturated fats are associated with heart disease because fatty deposits can build up in the body's blood vessels and slow down blood flow; polyunsaturates, being more liquid, are less likely to do this – hence the health claims.

We refer to 'fats' as those that are solid at room temperature, and 'oils' as those that are liquid. Fat that comes from animals is almost always a 'fat'; that which come from plants is almost always an 'oil'. This is because plants construct unsaturated fats, while animals can only synthesize saturated fats. Animals can only get energy by eating it, and so need a concentrated storage medium. Fat is that medium. Excess energy is converted to fat and stored until it is needed. The human body is especially efficient at this task.

Alcohol

Alcohol is also a nutrient, in that it provides energy and contains calories. One gram of pure alcohol produces about 7 calories, which the body can and does utilize as an energy source. The alcohol in 100 ml of 70-proof whisky has about 200 calories. Alcohol is not a fat, nor a carbohydrate, nor a protein, but behaves like a fat in some respects and like a carbohydrate in others.

Food Combining

A good diet should probably take about one third (37 per cent) of its calories from (mostly complex, or starchy) carbohydrates, one third (30 per cent) from protein, and one third (33 per cent) from fat (mostly polyunsaturated).

In practice, this 37/30/33 ratio is far from perfect. The basic idea, if you're trying to lose weight, is to reduce the amount of fat you take in, replacing its calories with other sources of energy. Fat, *per se*, has few vitamins and minerals, though vitamins A and D are important exceptions. Fat is chiefly only calories.

You also need to pay attention to the different sources of carbohydrate. Sugars provide the quickest source of energy, which is why glucose tablets and drinks are so useful when you feel exhausted, but many sugary snacks are also 'empty carbodrates' in that they *only* provide energy and none of the other essential nutrients. A slimmer should always seek foods that deliver additional nutritional benefits besides pure energy. If you eat too many snacks to satisfy an immediate hunger, the excess may get converted into fat. Starch gets converted into energy more slowly, and a few starchy foods – bread, pasta, root vegetables, beans, cereals – also contain other important nutrients and fibre.

Fat Conversion

Not all bodies are equally good at converting excess energy into fat. Let's put it another way – some people are prone to fatness and some are not. Two people can eat identically sized meals; one will evacuate all that is not required and one will store the excess as fat – around the stomach if he is a man, around the hips and thighs if she is a woman. There is no real 'explanation' for this. And there aren't just these two types of people, there is a progressive scale between those who are essentially 'thinnies' and those who are 'fatties'. It is the 'fatties', of course, who have to be more concerned with calorie control. They have got one clear advantage over 'thinnies', though: a thin person who suffers from a long illness will usually take longer to achieve full recovery than a fat one, because there are less fat reserves to draw upon.

There is one other feature about how fat is stored in the body that is critical to understanding the problems of weight control. A fat cell in the body is composed of one part of fat to 4 to 5 parts water. This explains why 'it is so hard to take off, so easy to put on': 10 grams of solid 'energy food' taken in and then stored as fat may show up as 50 or 60 grams of added body weight. It also explains why the first week of a diet always seems to produce extremely good results – you are losing the trapped water.

What You Should Weigh

These are average tables, with figures in pounds and kilograms. Although you may be more used to thinking in terms of pounds, you'll find calculations are easier if you switch to kilograms.

The figures have been derived from tables produced by life assurance companies; allowance has been made for the fact that some of us have bigger frames, broader shoulders, stockier builds and heavier bones than others. Be honest with yourself, though, and try and visualize what you'd like your body to look like. There is also an instant 'skin-fold' test you can try to see if you are carrying excess weight: stand naked in front of a mirror and see how big a fold of flesh you can pinch out from your tummy area or your buttocks or thighs. If the fold is more than 3 cm (just over an inch) without causing any tautening of surrounding flesh – you are carrying extra weight.

How to Weigh Yourself

- Always use the same scales.
- Weigh yourself at the same time of day. Most people wait until their stomach is empty, but whatever you do keep to one pattern. Your lowest weight of the day is usually first thing in the morning.
- Wear more or less the same clothes each time. (The tables assume you are wearing 2 to 3 kilograms – 5 to 6lb of clothing).
- Use the scales properly. Make sure they are firmly set on an even floor and read zero when no one is standing on them. Stand with your weight evenly distributed.

Men: desirable weights in outdoor clothing

Height Ft in/cm	Small Frame lb/kg	Medium Frame lb/kg	Large Frame lb/kg
5'2/158	112–120/50.5–54.5	118–129/53.5–58.5	126–141/57.0–64.0
5'3/160	115–123/52.0–56.0	121–133/55.0–60.5	129–144/58.5–65.0
5'4/163	118–128/53.5–57.0	124–136/56.0–62.0	132–148/60.0–67.0
5'5/165	121–129/55.0–58.5	127–139/57.5–63.0	135–152/61.0–67.0
5'6/168	124–133/56.0–60.5	130–143/58.5–65.0	138–156/62.5–71.0
5'7/170	128–137/58.0–62.0	134–147/61.0–66.5	142–161/64.5–73.0
5'8/173	132–141/60.0–64.0	138–152/64.5–71.0	147–166/66.5–75.5
5'9/175	136–145/62.0–66.0	142–156/64.5–71.0	151–170/68.5–77.0
5'10/178	140–150/63.5–68.0	146–160/66.0–72.5	155–174/70.0–79.0
5'11/180	144–154/65.0–70.0	150–165/68.0–75.0	159–179/72.0–81.0
6'0/183	148–158/67.0–71.5	154–170/70.0–77.0	164–184/74.5–83.5
6'1/185	152–162/69.0–73.5	158–175/71.5–79.0	168–189/76.0–85.5
6'2/188	156–167/71.0–76.0	162–180/73.5–81.5	173–194/78.5–88.0
6'3/190	160–171/72.5–77.5	167–185/76.0–84.0	178–199/80.5–90.5
6'4/193	164–175/74.5–79.0	172–190/78.0–86.0	182–204/82.5–92.5

Women: desirable weights in outdoor clothing

Height Ft in/cm	Small Frame lb/kg	Medium Frame lb/kg	Large Frame lb/kg
5'2/158	112–120/50.5–54.5	118–129/53.5–58.5	126–141/57.0–64.0
5'3/160	115–123/52.0–56.0	121–133/55.0–60.5	129–144/58.5–65.0
5'4/163	118–128/53.5–57.0	124–136/56.0–62.0	132–148/60.0–67.0
5'5/165	121–129/55.0–58.5	127–139/57.5–63.0	135–152/61.0–67.0
5'6/168	124–133/56.0–60.5	130–143/58.5–65.0	138–156/62.5–71.0
5'7/170	128–137/58.0–62.0	134–147/61.0–66.5	142–161/64.5–73.0
5'8/173	132–141/60.0–64.0	138–152/64.5–71.0	147–166/66.5–75.5
5'9/175	136–145/62.0–66.0	142–156/64.5–71.0	151–170/68.5–77.0
5'10/178	140–150/63.5–68.0	146–160/66.0–72.5	155–174/70.0–79.0
5'11/180	144–154/65.0–70.0	150–165/68.0–75.0	159–179/72.0–81.0
6'0/183	148–158/67.0–71.5	154–170/70.0–77.0	164–184/74.5–83.5
6'1/185	152–162/69.0–73.5	158–175/71.5–79.0	168–189/76.0–85.5
6'2/188	156–167/71.0–76.0	162–180/73.5–81.5	173–194/78.5–88.0
6'3/190	160–171/72.5–77.5	167–185/76.0–84.0	178–199/80.5–90.5
6'4/193	164–175/74.5–79.0	172–190/78.0–86.0	182–204/82.5–92.5

Kilograms, Stones and Pounds

Kg	Stones	lb	Kg	Stones	lb
41.4	6.5	91	85.9	13.5	189
44.6	7.0	98	89.1	14.0	196
47.3	7.5	105	92.3	14.5	203
50.9	8.0	112	95.5	15.0	210
54.1	8.5	119	98.6	15.5	217
57.3	9.0	126	101.8	16.0	224
60.5	9.5	133	105.0	16.5	231
63.6	10.0	140	108.2	17.0	238
66.8	10.5	147	111.4	17.5	245
70.0	11.0	154	114.6	18.0	252
73.2	11.5	161	117.7	18.5	259
76.4	12.0	168	120.9	19.0	266
79.6	12.5	175	124.1	19.5	273
82.7	13.0	182	127.3	20.0	280

Taking a Look at Your Lifestyle

Before you can set yourself dietary targets you need to analyse a few things: In the first place, you need to know how much energy you use up during the day.

How Much Energy Does Your Body Use?

Using tables, nutritionists can work our fairly accurately the precise amount of energy you need to function during your normal day.

First, so much is needed simply to keep your body alive, even if you are doing no more than lying in bed staring at the ceiling. This figure is called either your *Resting Energy Requirement* or your *Basal Metabolic Rate*. The table below shows the resting energy requirement for various people. Here are some averages:

	Weight (kg)	kcal /hr	kcal /day
Infant, 1 year old	10	21	500
Child, 8 years old	25	42	1000
Adult female	55	54	1300
Adult male	65	67	1600

Now, a more accurate figure, based on any weight – multiply this figure by your weight in kilograms:

	kcal /kg/hr	kcal /kg/day
Infant	2.1	50
Child	1.6	40
Adult – male and female	1.0	24

Second, here are figures for the average amount of energy one would use during various sorts of activity during the day. They are based on someone weighing 65kg. If you weigh a little more you could expect to use a little more energy, if you weigh under 65kg your body would need a little less. The figures in the left-hand column are expressed in calories-per-hour, the right-hand column gives the rate for 10 minutes of an activity.

Activity	Cal/hr	Cal/10 min
Aerobics, average	430	72
Circuit-training	510	85
Climbing stairs	660	110
Cycling, racing	660	110
Cycling, relaxed	240	40
Cycling, uphill	600	100
Dancing, fast	410	68
Dancing, relaxed	380	63
Driving a car	120	20
Gardening, digging	480	80
Gardening, weeding	210	35
Golf	390	65
Hill-climbing	480	80
Hill-climbing with a back-pack	510	85
Horse-riding, moderate	100	17
Horse-riding, trot	300	50
House-cleaning	240	40
Knitting	90	15
Playing piano	150	25
Running, fast	400	67
Running, slow	280	47
Running, medium jogging	330	55
Shopping	240	40
Sitting	90	15
Skiing	390	65
Sleeping	60	10
Squash	840	140
Swimming, fast	600	100
Swimming, relaxed	510	85
Tennis	420	70
Typing	120	20
Walking, normal	240	40
Walking, quickly	360	60
Weight training	420	70
Work, heavy manual	450	75
Work, light industrial	240	40
Work, moderately heavy	400	67
Writing	120	20

Once you have some idea of how much energy you burn in a given day, you must next add up the calorific value of the food you normally eat during the course of your day. But there is a third factor: you also need to know *when* you eat.

When Do You Eat?

In these days of snacks and 'eating-on-demand' it is important to keep track of your eating habits. You need to be aware of your patterns of *hunger* and *appetite*. Hunger is when your body demands to be fed, appetite is about your taste preferences.

Our changed lifestyle patterns mean that the times we feel hungry may be quite unexpected. If we find ourselves eating both when our bodies send us pangs of hunger and on those occasions when social conventions expect us to – traditional meal times, in other words – our calorie intake is likely to go up dramatically. In addition, if we haven't identified the times of the day when we are likely to feel hungry, we have almost no chance of developing a properly disciplined calorie-controlled diet.

Here are some examples of the new 'snacking' lifestyles and the implications for calorie intake. The examples shown here are for people who are not on any sort of diet:

Stay-at-home mother, one pre-school child, one child in education, partner with 'regular' job

	kcal
early morning tea	70
breakfast	680
snack after returning from taking older child to school	110
elevenses during shopping	410
munching during lunch preparation	80
lunch	470
snack while feeding younger child	110

snack with older child on its return from school	110
munching during evening meal preparation	90
evening meal with partner	790
late night snack	120
	2940

Executive who travels a great deal

early morning coffee	70
on-road breakfast	870
coffee and biscuits during first visit	190
coffee and biscuits during second visit	230
lunch	1130
tea and biscuits during third visit	190
snack during petrol fill-up	460
tea during fourth visit	70
early evening drink·and snack	420
evening meal	1070
late evening snack	120
	4820

Factory worker on afternoon shift

early morning tea and toast	310
late breakfast	680
elevenses	230
lunch	1020
arrival at work snack	90
late afternoon snack	130
arrival at home snack	120
evening meal	980
late evening snack	120
	3680

If you think these calculations are exaggerated, think again: for the most part the size of the main meal has been adjusted downwards to allow for the increase in the number of snacks.

Your body, like any other machine, should be fuelled shortly before it is expected to work. For this reason it is far better to eat a good, nourishing and energy-giving breakfast, give it a few minutes to digest, and let that take you through the morning. If you are on a slimming diet, you will find there is far less temptation to have mid-morning snacks. Almost certainly the foods that make up breakfast (cereal, orange juice, tea or coffee) are far more nourishing overall and far less full of calories weight-for-weight than the sugary and starchy materials that make up so many small snacks. If at all possible, your lunch and evening meals should be about the same size. The lunch should keep you going throughout the afternoon and the evening meal should be designed to do no more than prevent hunger pains from keeping you awake at night. If you concentrate most of your day's eating into the evening, too much food energy will get absorbed into your body while you sleep and, instead of being put to work immediately, it will start the chemical process which converts it into deposits of fat.

The best pattern of all, from the standpoint of your metabolism, is frequent (low-calorie) 'snacking' – but no main meals. Each snack should be around 200 calories, and afterwards there should be an opportunity for proper digestion – no eating on the run. But the snacks have to provide a balanced and complete diet, and that might not be particularly easy.

There is another reason for examining your eating habits. If you are too fat, you will almost certainly find that you have developed a strong preference for foods that will carry on making you fat. You must change your tastes, if only gradually. You must wean your taste buds off the high-calorie foods they may at present prefer.

The Calorie Tables

The calorie listings in this book attempt to use a scheme which is practical for the reader rather than going all out for 'scientific' consistency.

Most food is – still – basically a natural product. For this reason the actual energy and nutritional value of a given dish may vary from what the tables suggest. The amount of sugar in fruit increases as it ripens; the amount of fat in meat increases as the animal grows older. Recipes for the same dish may vary slightly. Even for such standard items as regular pasteurized milk an examination of the cartons sold by the UK's leading supermarkets will show that the energy content varies slightly. So: treat all the values given here as almost, rather than completely, accurate.

Within each category a representative range has been selected – clearly it was impossible to include every food, every way to cook a food and every brand-name product. This would make for a great deal of pointless repetition. In a typical large UK supermarket you could expect to find up to 3000 'own brand' food items. For each of these there will be at least three or four competitors from named producers, but in some cases there may be twenty. And there are, depending on how you count them up, nine or ten major UK supermarket chains.

In the tables you should find all the basic foods and ingredients plus a wide range of less popular 'generic' foods. A 'generic' ingredient or dish is one not sold by brand name. 'Wholemeal bread' is a generic name; 'Hovis' is a brand. The listings include a wide range of branded products but concentrate on the brand-leaders and others that are somehow typical.

For convenience, the tables have been arranged into a series of broad categories – bread, fruit, fish, meat, and so on. However, with the increase in the range of 'just heat it up' food products, it is becoming increasingly difficult to decide where to place them – is the best home for a supermarket's own-brand version of chill-cooked lasagne pescatori in Pasta, Fish or Recipe Dishes, for example? Again, similar foods appear in a variety of packs and 'finishes' – fresh, frozen, chilled, canned – and these days they can be displayed almost anywhere in a supermarket. Judging by the organization of the dietary information material sent to us by the leading UK supermarkets, they have no definitive answers either. This means you may have to look in more than one place in the book to find the food in which you are immediately interested.

The inclusion of one branded product rather than another or one from a particular supermarket 'own-brand' range doesn't imply some hidden quality test. The aim has been to provide a sufficient range so that you can guess at the calorific values of almost anything you are likely to come across. Occasionally different brands are included to make a point – either that apparently dissimilar items have the same calorific value, or that dishes sold under almost identical names may have been made from quite a wide variety of recipes and hence display a surprising range of energy contents.

Generic items are usually quoted in kilocalories per 100 grams (kcal/100g), make it easy to compare different sorts of food. 100 grams is about 3.5 imperial ounces. Fluids are quoted in kcal/100 ml (millilitres) – that is one tenth of a litre, 3.5 fluid ounces or 0.175 of an imperial pint. (A US pint is 16 fluid ounces compared to the imperial's 20 fluid ounces. 1 millilitre, is the same as 1 cubic centimetre, cc.) Where it helps there may also be calculations for individual portions, but people's views vary on what constitutes a reasonable-sized portion.

Bear in mind that many foods contain inedible elements such as bone, skin or pips. You should compare our suggestions with what you actually put on a plate. Remember also that some items may need reconstituting with water before you eat them and this will drastically change the calorific value per 100 grams. In fact, any form of cooking will change the calorific value per 100 grams, either by adding water or, as in the case of toasting, by removing it. There may be other changes as well, such as converting inedible carbohydrate into an eatable form, or adding sugar to taste.

Branded items may also be quoted using these measurements, but in many cases it is more useful to quote by pack or portion size, as that is what you will actually be eating. In some cases food manufacturers have not given all the information we would have liked; as a result, inconsistencies in their labelling information are sometimes reflected in the tables.

Methods of Weight Control

Under normal conditions we are used to a varied and interesting range of foods. In fact, quite apart from the considerations of weight, it is only by having a varied diet that we can be sure to have the right mixture and quantities of all the other nutrients our bodies need. An ideal weight-reducing diet retains this variety, but reduces the incidence of high energy content foods – indeed, if permanent results are wanted, you should hardly realize that you are on a diet.

The first thing to do is consult your doctor. He or she will check over your medical history to ensure that the reason for your over-weight is simply over-consumption and not some more serious underlying condition. You must also see your doctor if you are pregnant or have recently had a child. Similarly if you have had or think you may have a heart condition, do not diet without medical advice. Plump children who have become much too fat for their own good must also let the doctor determine the best course of action.

The Low-Calorie Diet

This is the most basic and reliable plan available. You set yourself a given energy intake for each day (measured in calories) and stick to it until you reach your target weight. When you are your ideal size you then increase your calorie intake to just the level to keep your body fuelled throughout its day's activities.

There are two targets to go for: the 1500-calorie and 1000-calorie limits. The 1500-calorie plan is best suited to you if:

- you are used to big meals and would be inclined to cheat if you had less to eat;
- you lead a relatively active physical life;
- you have a great deal of weight to lose and need to pace your slimming carefully if you are to have any success.

The 1000-calorie plan is better if:
- you can cope with the idea of fairly small meals;
- you lead a reasonably passive life;
- your overall weight reduction programme is to lose no more than 15 kilos.

Don't try to go below the 1000 calorie limit.

You can of course set a 1200- or 1400-daily calorie level instead. On a daily 1200-calorie diet you should lose fat at the rate of about 1 per cent of your total body weight each week.

The psychological back-up you use is up to you. Some people are very self-disciplined and can keep a mental note of all the calories they have taken in. Others find it useful to keep a little notebook or diary. Others need the support of friends and family – or the confessional surroundings of 'Weight Watcher'-type groups where you are expected to 'tell' of any transgressions.

Other Diet Schemes

Some people prefer other dieting methods. Here are two frequently-touted alternatives.

The Low-carbohydrate Diet. The idea here is to count carbohydrates instead of calories – typically you are urged to limit yourself to 50 grams of carbohydrate a day. 50 grams of carbohydrate provides about 200 calories. Many foods contain no carbohydrate, and it is assumed that, by limiting your intake of carbohydrate, your intake of the other energy-providing ingredients will come up to somewhere between 1000 and 1500 calories a day. The advantage of the scheme is that there are fewer figures to manipulate and so the arithmetic is easier. The drawback is that the calculations can deceive. 50 grams of Cheddar cheese, the amount you might have with a cheese salad, contains no carbohydrate but has 12.7 grams of protein and 17.3 grams of fat – and will account for more than 200 calories!

The No-count Diet. This diet involves no counting, merely learning lists. It is easy but also very inflexible and likely to become increasingly inaccurate the longer a diet plan is supposed to last.

In Category 1 of this diet are foods you can eat as much of as you like: meat, poultry, game, fish, eggs, green vegetables, a few root vegetables, some fresh fruit, salads, and unsweetened tea or coffee. Category 2 is made up of foods to be eaten only in moderate quantities: milk, cheese, fresh fruit (the sweeter varieties), peas, beans, carrots, parsnips, etc., cream, butter, margarine and fats. The third category of foods are never (or only very rarely) to be eaten: sugar, sweets, chocolate, candy, alcohol, soft drinks, cakes and pastries, jam and marmalade, syrups, tinned fruit, crisps, nuts, fried foods, potatoes, pasta, bread and breakfast cereals.

Slimming Foods

There is no such thing as a 'slimming food' – one that will make you lose weight. Calorie-reduced prepackaged foods are usually traditional recipes made with low-calorie ingredients – bulky vegetables will be used instead of potatoes or rice, the 'mayonnaise' will be based on fromage frais, skimmed milk or processed whey rather than egg, lemon juice and oil, etc. There are also an increasing number of oil and fat substitutes, such as modified carbohydrates, dextrins, polyglycerolesters, polysaccharides, *Simplesse* from *NutraSweet* (an egg protein/milk protein/sugar product), oil/cereal/protein formulations, combinations of dextrin or protein with sucrose polyesters, carboxylate esters, polycarboxylic acid esters, esterified propoxylated glycerol and polysiloxanes. Whatever else they are, these new products are in no way 'natural'!

The most common artificial sweetener used to be saccharin, which can sometimes have a slightly bitter undertaste. These days increasing use is made of aspartame (NutraSweet), which has a much more acceptable taste.

Starch-reduced foods include certain breads, rolls and crisp breads. Special flour is used which enables more air to be pumped into the risen dough. The result is bread which looks as bulky as ordinary bread but weighs rather less.

Food bulkers are branded slimmers' foods which usually contain a fair amount of cellulose, so the stomach feels full without any calories being added. Some brands contain additional minerals and vitamins to overcome the problem of nutritional deficiency. You may also find 'quack' ingredients – herbs and the like for which unsubstantiated claims are made. Occasionally you will also find brands with laxatives in them – partly to counteract the constipation these diet foods can create and partly, it is alleged, to stop the stomach from retaining 'unnecessary' food. Laxatives should only be used under medical supervision or very occasionally and should not be part of any daily diet.

A few people do seem to find these 'slimming foods' useful, but many more get on perfectly well without them. They are usually very expensive in terms of what you get. Sometimes the very cost is supposed to be part of the 'treatment' – an added incentive to get the weight off and the diet over with!

There are also products available in some health food shops which are borderline drugs. Because they are technically 'food' they are subject to none of the important regulations which control the way in which medicines are offered for sale to the public. Nevertheless some of these products have very powerful and unexpected effects. There really are no safe short-cuts to controlling your weight; a 'natural' label doesn't make a dangerous quasi-pharmaceutical any safer.

Slimming Medicines
Do not use pills or other medicines unless prescribed for you by your doctor. Do not hunt around for doctors attached to special slimming clinics in the hope that they will give you miracle drugs that your own doctor would refuse to prescribe.

There are three sorts of medication sometimes suggested; the less reputable type of clinic sometimes offers pill cocktails, the blend being much more powerful than the individual constituents by themselves:

1. Drugs to make your stomach feel full; often bulking agents.
2. Fat-reducing drugs – sometimes pills, sometimes hormone injections.
3. Amphetamines. These make you feel less hungry and very energetic. They carry very unfortunate risks, including addiction or habituation and also other psychological side-effects.

The best method of weight control is the one that works – safely and permanently. A calorie-controlled diet should not be a temporary device to get you back to a 'normal' weight; it is for life.

Bread

Fresh bread is 50 per cent carbohydrate. Nearly all this carbohydrate is in the form of starch, with sugars making up 2 to 4 per cent, depending on the recipe. Bread also contains 8 per cent protein, 2 per cent fat and 40 per cent water.

Toasting has the effect of reducing the water content in bread by about 20 per cent.

By the time bread has been fried it consists of only 8 per cent water; the energy nutrients then become: 8 per cent protein, 30 per cent fat and approximately 50 per cent carbohydrate.

Some bread doughs, for example those used for croissants, Indian naan and the Jewish cholla, have much higher levels of fat, which may have been introduced into the recipe either as butter or oil.

Apart from those doughs which contain significant amounts of fat, there is no cholesterol in bread.

Brown breads and those with added fibre are not, weight for weight, significantly lower in calorie than white bread, though of course they have other health benefits.

Crisp breads have had much of the water removed – typically they are under 10 per cent water as opposed to the 40 per cent in regular bread.

'Slimmer's Breads' usually have additional quantities of air or gas pumped into the dough during the baking process. The bulking up, of course, is supposed to induce the slimmer to eat less.

Effects of 'spreads': this is how you calculate the calorific value of a slice of bread or toast together with butter, margarine, jam, etc. (in grams):

- A 'thick' slice of pre-sliced bread is usually 40 to 45 g, a 'thin' slice is 25 g. If you cut your own bread, a thin slice will be about 40 g and a thick slice 50 to 55 g.
- A typical 'large' slice will carry 12 to 15 g of butter or butter-like spread: 90–110 calories of butter, about the same for margarine, and 45–55 for a low-fat spread. A typical coating of jam or marmalade would be 15 g, around 40 calories; a reduced-sugar jam would be 20 calories.
- A typical thick piece of toast (from a pre-sliced loaf) with butter and jam would be 250 calories – but, if the coatings were generous, it could be up to 330 calories. Two thin slices, each with the standard amount of butter and jam (or marmalade) would account for 400 calories!
- Most people put more butter/margarine on very fresh bread and on toast which is still hot.

Food Category or Brand	Calories /100g	Portion	Size /g	Calories /port
Generic Breads				
bagel	270			
brioche	370			
brown	218			
brown rolls, crusty	255			

Food Category or Brand	Calories /100g	Portion	Size /g	Calories /port
brown rolls, soft	268			
brown, toasted	272			
chapatis, with fat	328			
chapatis, without fat	202			
cholla	393			
ciabatta	259			
croissant	360			
currant bread	289			
currant bread, toasted	323			
French stick	270			
granary	235			
hamburger bun	264			
malt bread	268			
naan bread	336			
poppadums, fried	369			
pitta, white	265			
rye bread	219			
Vitbe	229			
white loaf	235			
white roll, crusty	280			
white roll, soft	268			
white, fried in lard	503			
white, fried in oil	503			
white, sliced	217			
white, toasted	265			
wholemeal	215			
wholemeal roll	241			
wholemeal, toasted	252			

Branded Breads
Allinson

		Portion		Calories /port
100% wholemeal, meidium slice		1 slice		79
100% wholemeal, thick slice		1 slice		95
HiBran bread		1 slice		53
soft wholemeal		1 slice		67
stoneground, large		1 slice		79

Food Category or Brand	Calories /100g	Portion	Size /g	Calories /port
stoneground, small		1 slice		52
wholemeal rolls		1 roll		151
Asda				
baguette	241			
stoneground loaf		1 slice		84
white loaf, medium		1 slice		77
white loaf, thick		1 slice		93
wholemeal loaf		1 slice		66
wholemeal muffins		1 muffin		120
Rustique	236			
Co-op				
crispbreads		1 slice		25
crumpets		1 crumpet		80
soft white baps		1 bap		145
soft white rolls		1 roll		110
wholemeal baps		1 bap		120
Country Pride				
crushed wheat, white		1 slice		80
Danish white		1 slice		50
Danish toaster		1 slice		60
traditional white, large		1 slice		80
traditional white, small		1 slice		65
Hovis				
Hovis bread	212			
Hovis bread, toasted	271			
golden bran		1 slice		80
golden oatbran, large		1 slice		85
granary malted, large		1 slice		80
granary malted rolls		1 roll		140
granary malted, small		1 slice		65
high-fibre wholemeal		1 slice		80

Food Category or Brand	Calories /100g	Portion	Size /g	Calories /port
large white, medium slice		1 slice		75
large white, thick slice		1 slice		90
light wholemeal		1 slice		70
multi-grain, large		1 slice		80
organic stoneground, small		1 slice		60
stoneground wholemeal, large		1 slice		80
stoneground wholemeal, small		1 slice		60
wheatgerm, large		1 slice		85
wheatgerm, small		1 slice		65
wholemeal baps		1 bap		120
International Harvest				
croissants		1 croissant		185
mini croissants		1 croissant		145
mini white pitta		1 pitta		80
mini wholemeal pitta		1 pitta		70
naan		1 naan		390
white pitta		1 pitta		180
wholemeal pitta		1 pitta		160
Kingsmill				
large		1 slice		80
rolls		1 roll		125
small		1 slice		65
Mighty White				
rolls		1 roll		230
softgrain		1 slice		80
Mothers Pride				
Big T white		1 slice		115
brown baps		1 bap		140
burger buns		1 bun		140
croissants		1 croissant		220
crumpets		1 crumpet		80

Food Category or Brand	Calories /100g	Portion	Size /g	Calories /port
Danish toaster		1 slice		65
Danish white		1 slice		50
light white		1 slice		55
long rolls		1 roll		110
morning rolls, white		1 roll		75
ploughman's rolls		1 roll		160
Scotch rolls		1 roll		130
Scottish batch		1 slice		120
traditional white, small		1 slice		65
white, long		1 slice		85
Nimble				
malty brown		1 slice		50
soft wholemeal		1 slice		50
white		1 slice		50
Safeway				
garlic baguette	305			
soft grain bread	224			
(medium & thick cut)				
traditional wholemeal bread				
rolls	217			
wholemeal baps	240			
wholemeal bread	232			
(medium & thick)				
wholemeal pitta breads	219			
(mini & standard)				
Sainsbury's				
all butter croissants		each		188
brown		slice		72
crumpets		each		75
Danish		slice		51
economy wholemeal		slice		72
garlic baguette		each		594

Food Category or Brand	Calories /100g	Portion	Size /g	Calories /port
granary malted wholemeal		thick slice		96
home bake baguette		each		316
malted brown granary		slice		82
mini all butter croissants		each		140
mini pitta, white		each		89
muffins		each		173
nature's Choice wholemeal		slice		49
pitta, white		each		165
soft grain		slice		82
stoneground wholemeal		slice		72
teacakes		each		171
wheatgerm hovis		slice		61
white floury batch		per roll		156
white premium		slice		74
white, sliced baps		each		144
wholemeal		slice		77
wholemeal country rolls		per roll		152
wholemeal floury batch		per roll		141
wholemeal harvest grain		each		150

St Michael (Marks & Spencer)

baguette	181
brown rolls	275
brown soda bread	229
cheese bruschettine	430
ciabatta	262
cob loaf	235
crusty white rolls	181
garlic bread	380
granary rolls	261
high bran	210
Italian style ring bread	210
long life white medium	230
naan bread	332
oatmeal farmhouse	245
organic mixed seed loaf	261

Food Category or Brand	Calories /100g	Portion	Size /g	Calories /port
organic white rolls	246			
organic wholemeal sliced	198			
pitta	282			
soft grain (medium)	283			
soft oatmeal rolls	280			
sunflower/honey loaf	308			
white farmhouse	250			
white soft farmhouse	245			
Sunblest				
bloomer		1 slice		70
brown, long		1 slice		75
crusty cob		1 cob		150
Danish white		1 slice		40
farmhouse baps		1 bap		135
soft brown rolls		1 roll		120
soft white rolls		1 roll		115
split tin		1 slice		70
white, long		1 slice		80
Tesco				
baguette	235			
brown	217			
brown rolls	235			
ciabatta	267			
multigrain wholemeal	246			
naan bread	286			
pitta bread	227			
soft white rolls	241			
white	228			
white farmhouse	361			
wholemeal	214			
Waitrose				
bloomer	216			
brown rolls	253			

Food Category or Brand	Calories /100g	Portion	Size /g	Calories /port
ciabatta	226			
farmhouse	216			
Greek olive bread	306			
malted wheat brown sliced	233			
soft white	245			
white medium sliced	258			
white organic	246			
white pitta	260			
wholemeal	235			
wholemeal medium sliced	200			
wholemeal organic	220			
wholemeal with oats	200			

Branded Slimmers' Breads

Hovis

light wholemeal		1 slice		70

Mothers Pride

light white		1 slice		55

Slimcea

brown		1 slice		45
white		1 slice		45

Tesco

white	247			
wholemeal	211			

Weight Watchers

brown or white		1 slice		30
brown or white rolls		1 roll		100
Danish brown		1 slice		40
Danish white		1 slice		45

Food Category or Brand	Calories /100g	Portion	Size /g	Calories /port

Branded Crispbreads
Co-op

savoury wheat		each		25

Lyons

Krispen, rye		each		15
Krispen, standard		each		15
Slice-a-rice		each		25

Ry-King

brown		each		35
fibre plus		each		30
golden		each		35
wheat plus		each		50

Ryvita

brown		each		25
crackerbread		each		20
high-fibre		each		25
high-fibre crackerbread		each		15
original		each		25
sesame seed		each		30

Sainsbury's

crispbread (wholemeal rye)		each		26
crisprolls		each		48
crissini Italian breadsticks		each		21
highland oatcakes		each		59
wheat & rye crackers		each		38
wholemeal bran biscuits		each		63
wholemeal krispwheat		each		17

Food Category or Brand	Calories /100g	Portion	Size /g	Calories /port
Branded Slimmers' Crispbreads				
Co-op				
light		each		25
Finn Crisp				
light rye		each		35
Gateway				
light		each		20
light wholemeal		each		15
Slymbread				
original		each		10
rye		each		10
sesame		each		15
wholemeal		each		10
Superdrug				
Supatrim light		each		20

Cakes and Biscuits

Cakes

A cake consists of between 50 and 70 per cent carbohydrate, 15 and 35 per cent water, 4 and 10 per cent protein and 5 and 30 per cent fat. The starch component of the carbohydrate may be as low as 8 per cent or as high as 30 per cent, and the sugars may vary from 30 per cent to 55 per cent.

Icing and cream fillings put up both the fat and sugar elements.

Depending on the recipe, the fats are principally either saturated or monounsaturated, with relatively low amounts of polyunsaturated.

Individual pastries covered in icing or sugar and with fillings, especially cream buns, will have the highest calorie count.

Biscuits

As for biscuits, most are 65–70 per cent carbohydrate, 5–10 per cent protein and 15–30 per cent fats. Coated and filled biscuits have a higher protein proportion of fat and a correspondingly lower proportion of protein. The highest proportion of fats will be saturated, though the amount varies from recipe to recipe.

Food Category or Brand	Calories /100g	Portion	Size /g	Calories /port
Generic Cakes				
battenburg	370	1 slice	80	296
cheesecake	492	1 slice	125	613
cherry cake	454	1 slice	125	565
chocolate cake	497	1 portion	100	497
coconut cakes	444	1 cake	80	355
cupcakes (iced)	356	1 cake	50	180
currant buns	305	1 bun	80	245
currant cake	418	1 portion	100	418
devil's food (iced)	337	1 portion	100	337
doughnuts	335	1 portion	100	335
Dundee cake	389	1 portion	100	389
Eccles cakes	518	1 cake	60	310
fruit cake	378	1 slice	125	470
ginger bread	381	1 slice	85	325
Madeira cake	393	1 slice	85	326
orange cake (iced)	469	1 slice	100	470
orange cake (plain)	465	1 slice	100	465
queens cakes	455	1 cake	75	315
rock cakes	419	1 cake	70	290
scones	369	1 scone	60	220
spongecake	308	1 slice	125	385
Swiss roll, chocolate	337	1 cake	75	253
Victoria sandwich	473	1 slice	125	590
Welsh cheesecake	489	1 cake	100	489

Branded Cakes

Asda

apple pie	378			
Bakewell slice	394			
battenburgh	440			

Food Category or Brand	Calories /100g	Portion	Size /g	Calories /port
chocolate fudge cake	377			
chocolate Swiss roll	364			
double chocolate cake	364			
Dundee	327			
fairy cakes	442			
lemon cake	392	1 slice		205
Madeira	390			
mini roll with jam & vanilla	350	1 roll		108
rich fruit	319			
sultana & cherry	353			

Cadbury's

SMALL CAKES

chocolate mini roll		1 roll		115
flake cake		1 cake		116
milk chocolate cake bars		1 cake		153
golden crisp cake bars		1 cake		175
jam mini roll		1 roll		113
caramel cake bar		1 cake		140

LARGE CAKES

chocolate cake	388			
chocolate roll	405	1 cake		232
Swiss gateau	420			

Lyons Bakery

SMALL CAKES

apple pie		1 pie		190
blackcurrant & apple pie		1 pie		200
caramel treat		1 cake		105
cherry Bakewell		1 cake		185
chocolate cupcake		1 cake		130
chocolate vanilla roll		1 roll		110
classic roll		1 roll		120
coconut crunch cake		1 cake		135

Food Category or Brand	Calories /100g	Portion	Size /g	Calories /port
farmhouse slice		1 cake		115
fruit puff		1 cake		95
golden midi roll		1 roll		140
iced tart		1 tart		155
jam tart		1 tart		140
lemon curd tart		1 tart		150
lemon meringue		1 cake		150
strawberry fancy		1 cake		125
sultana apple slice		1 cake		150
toffee cupcake		1 cake		125
trifle sponge		1 cake		75
LARGE CAKES				
battenburg	398			
chocolate Swiss roll	378			
raspberry Swiss roll	312			

Mr Kipling

SMALL CAKES				
almond slice		1 cake		132
apple & blackcurrant pie		1 pie		225
Bakewell slice		1 cake		137
caramel shortcake		1 cake		164
cherry Bakewell		1 cake		197
coconut macaroon		1 cake		97
French fancies		1 cake		104
Jaffa finger		1 cake		124
jam tart		1 tart		128
lemon slice		1 slice		133
mini battenburg cake		1 cake		126
mince slice		1 slice		163
strawberry sundae		1 cake		187
toffee apple tarts		1 cake		194

Food Category or Brand	Calories /100g	Portion	Size /g	Calories /port
LARGE CAKES				
Bakewell tart	418			
battenburg	398			
chocolate Swiss roll	378			
Dutch apple Bakewell	383			
fruit bake	356			
iced toffee tart	430			
lattice treacle tart	376			
Manor House	434			
pineapple soft fruit bake	331			
raspberry Swiss roll	312			
summer fruits dessert	372			

Sainsbury's

Food Category or Brand	Calories /100g	Portion	Size /g	Calories /port
SMALL CAKES				
all butter flapjack		per slice		149
bramley apple pie		per pie		242
cherry Bakewell		per cake		235
chocolate cupcake		per cake		134
chocolate mini roll		per roll		120
coconut Macaroon		per cake		142
Dutch apple turnover		per cake		138
economy apple pie		per tart		183
fondant fancy		per cake		103
jam tart		per tart		143
meringue nest		per nest		73
mince pie		per pie		165
LARGE CAKES				
Bakewell tart	418			
battenburg (large)	367			
choc Swiss roll	387			
Dundee	330			
Genoa	385			
ginger	344			

Food Category or Brand	Calories /100g	Portion	Size /g	Calories /port
iced fruit cake	346			
jam & buttercream Swiss roll	357			
lemon drizzle	353			
Madeira, lemon iced	396			
malt loaf	300			
sponge sandwich	145			
treacle tart	376			
walnut & coffee	440			

St Michael (Marks & Spencer)

angel cake	430			
apple sponge	283			
Bakewell tart	475			
banana loaf		each		400
battenburg	376			
blueberry muffin	335			
bramley apple pies	333			
carrot cake	350			
cherry cake	380			
chocolate brownie	440			
chocolate eclairs	418			
chocolate sponge roll	360			
chocolate Swiss roll	360			
double chocolate muffin	414			
Eccles cake	363			
egg custards	286			
flapjack	437			
fondant fancies	390			
iced finger bun	338			
iced sponge cake	400			
jam doughnut	300			
jam Swiss roll	285			
lemon sponge roll	340			
Madeira	405			
pain au chocolat	445			
rich fruit cake	365			

Food Category or Brand	Calories /100g	Portion	Size /g	Calories /port
sultana and cherry cake	370			
victoria sandwich	410			
viennese	495			

Sara Lee
chocolate fudge nut gateau		1 cake		1410

Tesco
SMALL CAKES

American muffin		1 cake		265
Belgian bun		1 bun		370
cherry Bakewell		1 cake		190
chocolate profiterole		1 cake		90
chocolate eclair		1 cake		330
corn crisp		1 cake		115
egg custard tart		1 tart		190
lemon curd tart		1 tart		160
sponge finger		1 cake		20

Waitrose
apple pies	357			
carrot & orange	350			
cherry Genoa	342			
chocolate chip	405			
chocolate Victoria sponge	430			
coconut choc fudge	443			
Eccles	382			
lemon iced Madeira	408			
mince pies	463			
paradise	381			
rich fruit	361			
strawberry cheesecake	309			
toffee	413			
walnut	408			

Food Category or Brand	Calories /100g	Portion	Size /g	Calories /port
Generic Biscuits				
chocolate digestive	493			
chocolate, full-coated	524			
cream crackers	440			
digestive	471			
flapjacks	484			
gingernut	456			
jaffa cakes	363			
oatcakes	441			
sandwich biscuits	513			
semi-sweet	457			
shortbread	498			
wafer, filled	535			
Asda				
cheese thin	532			
choc chip cookies	503			
custard creams	504			
digestive	493			
double chocolate creams	537			
fig rolls	377			
fruit shortcake	474			
fudge brownie dreams	477			
ginger nuts	447			
jaffa cakes	380			
malted milk	488			
milk chocolate digestive	512			
Nice biscuits	485			
rich tea	447			
shortcake	517			
Burton's				
Bourbon		1 biscuit		60
chocolate chip & hazelnut		1 biscuit		55
coconut		1 biscuit		50

Food Category or Brand	Calories /100g	Portion	Size /g	Calories /port
coconut cream		1 biscuit		60
coconut crisp		1 biscuit		35
coconut delight		1 biscuit		110
country snapjack		1 biscuit		80
fruit snapjack		1 biscuit		70
ginger nut		1 biscuit		45
jaffa cake		1 biscuit		40
Jammie Dodger		1 biscuit		85
Rich Tea		1 biscuit		45
shortcake		1 biscuit		50
strawberry cream		1 biscuit		60
Viscount		1 biscuit		90
Wagon Wheel		1 biscuit		167
Wagon Wheelie		1 biscuit		90

Cadbury's

Food Category or Brand	Calories /100g	Portion	Size /g	Calories /port
Bournville digestive		1 biscuit		45
butter shortie		1 biscuit		45
chocolate orange digestive		1 biscuit		45
cookie		1 biscuit		50
hazelnut wafer		1 biscuit		45
orange cream		1 biscuit		80

Farmhouse

Food Category or Brand	Calories /100g	Portion	Size /g	Calories /port
chocolate fruit ginger		1 biscuit		75
chocolate shortbread		1 biscuit		75
coconut drop		1 biscuit		90
currant Shrewsbury		1 biscuit		65
farmhouse oat		1 biscuit		65
Melting Moment		1 biscuit		75
mild ginger		1 biscuit		75
shortbread		1 biscuit		145
Shrewsbury		1 biscuit		70
wholemeal square		1 biscuit		85

Food Category or Brand	Calories /100g	Portion	Size /g	Calories /port
Fox's				
Blackwells		1 biscuit		82
brambles		1 biscuit		92
brandy snap		1 biscuit		55
butter tea		1 biscuit		63
chocolate crunch cream		1 biscuit		73
coconut crunch cream		1 biscuit		74
crinkle crunch		1 biscuit		51
crinklé crunch chocolate		1 biscuit		57
finger cream		1 biscuit		52
ginger crunch cream		1 biscuit		74
ginger snap		1 biscuit		35
golden crunch cream		1 biscuit		74
milk chocolate classic		1 biscuit		66
sunbreaks		1 biscuit		34
treacle crunch cream		1 biscuit		74
McVities				
Abbey Crunch	479	1 biscuit		46
all butter shortbread	541	1 biscuit		77
Bandit	533	1 biscuit		115
Boaster, hazelnut & chocolate chip	549	1 biscuit		93
Boaster, raisin & chocolate	515	1 biscuit		88
Cheddars	540	1 biscuit		21
chocolate fudge Yo Yo	551	1 biscuit		131
chocolate Hob Nob creams	508	1 biscuit		73
digestive	496	1 biscuit		73
digestive creams	513	1 biscuit		73
fruit shortcake	496	1 biscuit		52
ginger nut creams	471	1 biscuit		47
ginger nuts	471	1 biscuit		47
Hob Nobs	484	1 biscuit		69
Hob Nob bar	523	1 biscuit		138
Hob Nob fruit & nut cookie	501	1 biscuit		84

Food Category or Brand	Calories /100g	Portion Size /g		Calories /port
Jaffa Cake	384	1 biscuit		48
Rich Tea	481	1 biscuit		37

Sainsbury's

all butter		per biscuit		43
all butter shortbread fingers		per biscuit		103
bourbon		per biscuit		61
choc chip cookies		per biscuit		57
crunch creams		per biscuit		74
custard creams		per biscuit		59
farmhouse Highland shortbread		per biscuit		109
fig roll		per biscuit		72
fruit shortcake		per biscuit		38
Garibaldi		per biscuit		33
ginger crunch cream		per biscuit		74
ginger snap		per biscuit		48
jaffa cakes		per biscuit		48
jam sandwich cream		per biscuit		74
malted milk		per biscuit		39
milk choc digestive		per biscuit		86
milk choc rich tea		per biscuit		52
milk choc wafers		per wafer		45
pink wafer sandwich		per wafer		30
rich tea		per biscuit		43
thick plain chocolate		per biscuit		127

St Michael (Marks & Spencer)

bourbon creams	485			
butter crunch creams	517			
choc chip	506			
custard creams	517			
digestive biscuits	510			
ginger snap	445			
golden crunch		each		72
jaffa cakes	405			
jam sandwich creams	492			
milk choc digestive	522			

Food Category or Brand	Calories /100g	Portion	Size /g	Calories /port
milk cookie	484			
oatcakes	445			
plain choc digestive	518			
rich tea	460			
rich tea finger	471			
shortbread fingers	510			
white cookie	490			

Waitrose

bourbon	499			
choc brownie biscuit	542			
choc orange cookies	500			
custard creams	517			
digestive sweetmeal	502			
Garibaldi	389			
ginger cookies	476			
Nice biscuits	446			
rich tea	454			
shortcake	512			
treacle cookies	505			

Walkers

chocolate chip hazelnut		1 biscuit		90
hazelnut round		1 biscuit		95
honey & oatmeal		1 biscuit		85
muesli		1 biscuit		80
shortbread round		1 biscuit		90
stem ginger shortbread		1 biscuit		70
sultana		1 biscuit		80
treacle		1 biscuit		90

Cereals

The most popular breakfast cereals are made from corn, oats, wheat or rice, which are then heavily processed. Almost the entire energy content is in the form of carbohydrate and sugars. In the case of some of the cereal products aimed at children, over a third of the weight of the dried product is added sugar.

Mueslis and other cereals containing nuts will contain significant amounts of vegetable fat, up to 9 or 10 per cent. The deluxe (and hence more expensive) mueslis have more nuts and thus end up, weight for weight, with higher calorific values. Swiss-style mueslis may contain dried skimmed milk or whey powder.

Granolas are based on crunchy oats; the crunchiness comes from sugar-roasting the oats in oil, and this is why their calorific value is so high – the sugar content may be the equivalent of more than three teaspoons-full!

The figures given below are for the dry products. Assuming the addition of just under half a pint of regular milk, you will be adding a further 60 calories per serving; if you use skimmed milk, the addition will be about 30 calories, with semi-skimmed it will be about 40 calories; if you sprinkle on a couple of tablespoons of sugar, you are adding a further 100 to 120 calories.

Cereal bars are listed in the **Sugar, Syrups, Confectionery and Cereal Bars** section.

Food Category or Brand	Calories /100g	Portion	Size /g	Calories /port
Branded Cereals				
Allinson				
Bran Muesli	328	1 serving	30	98
Bran Plus	219	1 serving	30	66
Breakfast Muesli	354	1 serving	30	106
Asda				
bran flakes	331			
choco flakes	371			
cinnamon apple oat squares	389			
corn flakes	367			
crispy nut cornflakes	386			
frosted flakes	367			
fruit and fibre	374			
ready oats	356			
sultana bran	320			
Swiss style muesli	369			
Co-op				
chocolate chip muesli	404	1 serving	30	121
frosted cornflakes	393	1 serving	30	118
honey nut flakes	396	1 serving	30	119
Swiss-style muesli	389	1 serving	30	117
wheatflakes	364	1 serving	30	109
wholewheat muesli	379	1 serving	30	114

Food Category or Brand	Calories /100g	Portion	Size /g	Calories /port
Holland & Barrett				
original muesli	351	1 serving	30	105
apricot muesli	285	1 serving	30	86
fruit muesli	327	1 serving	30	98
nut muesli	359	1 serving	30	108
Jordan's				
Country Crisp with Raisins & Almonds	415	1 serving	50	208
Country Crisp with Raspberries	435	1 serving	50	218
Original Crunchy with Fruit	442	1 serving	50	221
Original Crunchy with Raisins	424	1 serving	50	213
Kellogg's				
All Bran Bite Size	290	1 serving	30	88
All Bran Buds	270	1 serving	30	82
All Bran Plus	270	1 serving	30	96
Chocolate Crispix	380	1 serving	30	114
Coco Pops	380	1 serving	30	114
Cornflakes	370	1 serving	30	111
Corn Pops	380	1 serving	30	114
Crunchy Nut Cornflakes	390	1 serving	30	117
Frosted Wheats	340	1 serving	30	102
Frosties	380	1 serving	30	114
Fruit 'n' Fibre	350	1 serving	30	105
Healthwise Bran Flakes	320	1 serving	30	96
Healthwise Oat Bran Flakes	350	1 serving	30	105
Healthwise Sultana Bran	320	1 serving	30	96
Honey Crispix	380	1 serving	30	114
Honey Loops	370	1 serving	30	111
Just Right	360	1 serving	30	108
Multi-Grain Start	360	1 serving	30	108
Raisin Wheats	320	1 serving	30	96
Rice Krispies	380	1 serving	30	114

Food Category or Brand	Calories /100g	Portion	Size /g	Calories /port
Ricicles	380	1 serving	30	114
Special K	370	1 serving	30	111
Sustain	360	1 serving	30	108

Quaker

Bran & Apple	425	1 serving	30	128
Oat Krunchies	383	1 serving	30	115
Puffed Wheat	328	1 serving	30	98
Quaker Oats	368	1 serving	30	110
Sultanas & Raisins	446	1 serving	30	134
Harvest Crunch	459	1 serving	30	137

Safeway

bran flakes	324			
choc & strawberry crunch	462			
coco crunchies	375			
corn flakes	367			
crispy malty flakes	361			
crunchy cereal	459			
fibre bran	276			
frosted flakes	373			
fruit & fibre	360			
golden puffs	375			
honey & nut corn flakes	394			
instant hot oat cereal	356			
luxury fruit & nut muesli	373			
reduced fat crunchy cereal	422			
rice crunchies	370			
savers muesli	358			
strudel porridge	348			
sultana bran	326			
Swiss style muesli	376			

Sainsbury's

bran flakes	324		30	156
coco snaps	372		30	170

Food Category or Brand	Calories /100g	Portion Size /g	Calories /port
cornflakes	367	30	169
fruit & fibre	354	30	165
honey nut cornflakes	338	30	175
hot oat cereal	391	30(150ml)	191
mini wheats	342	45	212
rice pops	370	30	105
sultana bran	320	30	155
Swiss style muesli	361	60	217
wholewheat biscuits	339	36(150ml)	191

(per portion values for cereals include 125 ml of semi-skimmed milk
except where stated)

St Michael (Marks & Spencer)

bran muesli	322
chocolate crunch	446
cornflakes	363
crunchy puffs	388
frosted flakes	365
quick porridge	398
strawberry cereal	455
Swiss style muesli	360
toffee & pecan	459

Tesco

bran flakes	336	1 serving	30	101
cocoa puffs	357	1 serving	30	107
corn flakes	343	1 serving	30	103
golden puffs	361	1 serving	30	108

Waitrose

branflakes	333
choc & hazelnut crunch	480
cornflakes	372
crisp rice	382
fruit & fibre	319

Food Category or Brand	Calories /100g	Portion	Size /g	Calories /port
fruit & nut muesli	367			
honey nut cornflakes	394			
luxury muesli	355			
oat crunchy almonds	396			
oat crunchy fruits	433			
porridge oats	392			
Swiss style muesli	364			

Weetabix

Alpen	365	1 serving	30	110
Alpen, no added sugar	357	1 serving	30	107
Alpen Nutty Crunch	381	1 serving	30	114
Alpen, tropical	379	1 serving	30	114
Weetabix	340	1 biscuit		64
Weetaflakes	368	1 serving	30	110
Weetos	384	1 serving	30	115

Crisps and Snacks

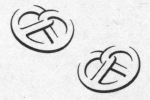

All crisp products have about the same calorific value, 500 kcal/100 g. Approximately 50 per cent of a true potato crisp is starch and almost 40 per cent will be fats; the rest is protein. In a low-fat potato crisp, the fat content will be around 20 per cent, though there is no formal definition of what 'low fat' means. For example, there is almost no calorific difference between Sainsbury's Crinkle Cut (i.e. normal) crisps and its low-fat range, but KP's low-fat range are just under 400 kcal/100 g, 100 calories less than its 'normal' crisps.

Many 'potato' crisps are made from specially processed potato as opposed to actual slices of raw potato, and many are actually made of processed corn (that is, maize). The presence of corn is obvious in items like tortilla chips, but less so in the various 'crackers' aimed at children, or the various pseudo-ethnic snacks from 'exotic' parts which may contain corn, processed potato and other flours.

'Mignons morceaux' are basically fried bread.

Many of these snacks contain significant amounts of salt – this may be important for people concerned with their blood-pressure.

Food Category or Brand	Calories /100g	Portion	Size /g	Calories /port
Branded Crisps				
Asda				
cheese & onion	530			
pickled onion	530			
prawn cocktail	530			
ready salted (lower fat)	481			
ready salted	553			
roast chicken	530			
salt and vinegar	524			
smoky bacon	530			
Boots Shapers				
bacon bites	431	bag	23	99
chargrilled chicken	482	bag	20	96
cheese and onion	482	bag	20	96
cheese puffs	492	bag	16	79
New York style salted pretzels	391	bag	24	92
prawn shells	469	bag	21	98
salt and vinegar crunchy sticks	456	bag	21	95
sea salt & black pepper	482	bag	20	96
sour cream chives	482	bag	20	96
Thai lemon lanterns	441	bag	18	80
tomato and herb twists	468	bag	20	93
Co-op				
cheese puffs	578	bag	50	289
chip snacks	482	bag	50	241
crisps (all flavours)	529	bag	25	132
onion rings	522	bag	50	261
Streaky Crispies	476	bag	50	238
Kettle Crisps				
lightly salted	496			
yoghurt & green onion	517			

Food Category or Brand	Calories /100g	Portion	Size /g	Calories /port
salsa & mesquite	491			
New York cheddar	483			

McCoy's
beef	518	bag		207
cheese	523	bag		209
original	528	bag		211

Pringles
light	511			
original	570			
sour cream & onion	571			

Sainsbury's
bacon crispies	473	bag	50	237
cheese savouries	534	bag	33	176
cornitos, bacon flavour		bag	35	167
crinkle cut (less than 25% fat)		bag	25	119
gourmet crisps	495			
original tortillas	477			
prawn crackers		bag	50	268
ready salted crisps		bag	25	134
salt & vinegar crisps		bag	25	131
savoury twirls with cheese		twirl		34

St Michael (Marks & Spencer)
cheese tasters	533			
handcooked balsamic vinegar	474			
handcooked ready salted	502			
handcooked salt/pepper crisps	498			
prawn crackers	516			
ready salted crinkle	474			
ready salted	543			

Food Category or Brand	Calories /100g	Portion	Size /g	Calories /port
salt and vinegar	529			
sour cream & chive	482			
spring onion	530			
Waitrose				
assorted flavours	545			
lower fat crinkles	496			
onion rings	475			
ready salted	560			
ready salted rings	519			
salt & vinegar crisps	560			
salt & vinegar twirls	467			
spicy Thai chips	478			

Dairy Products

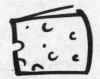

Milk

Milk is sometimes said to be the most nutritionally complete of all foods. Whole milk is 88 per cent water, 3 per cent protein, just under 5 per cent carbohydrate (in the form of sugars) and 4 per cent fat, two thirds of which is saturated fat.

In a *full skimmed milk* there is just a trace of fat, and the water proportion is 91 per cent. With *semi-skimmed milk* there is 1.6 per cent fat and just under 89 per cent water. Pasteurizing and homogenizing have no effects on any of these proportions, but in *sterilized milk*, some of the water content is lost.

In an *evaporated milk* the water content is down to 70 per cent, fat is up to 9 or 10 per cent, and protein and carbohydrate at about 8 per cent each.

Condensed milks are often sweetened. In condensed whole milk, the water content may be down as far as 25 per cent, fat at 10 per cent, but carbohydrate in the form of sugars up to 55 per cent.

Flavoured milks, for example with chocolate or fruit, will almost inevitably have additional carbohydrates in the form of sugars. There may also be additional fats.

Milk shakes are listed under **Drinks** (Non-alcoholic).

From a purely energy point-of-view, whole *goat's milk* is not significantly different from whole cow's milk.

The figures given for *dried milks* are for the undiluted powder and are rather misleading.

Soya milk isn't milk at all, but a liquid made from the soya bean. Other imitation milks are made from coconut oil and corn syrup.

Butter is listed in the **Fats and Oils** section.

Ice-cream has its own section.

Cream

Cream is the part of milk with the highest fat content. The main difference between the various creams offered for sale is the actual amount of fat.

Half cream has not less than 12 per cent fat and is almost 80 per cent water.

Single cream has at least 18 per cent fat.

Double cream is not less than 48 per cent fat.

Clotted cream is a minimum of 55 per cent fat and has the least amount of water – just over 30 per cent.

Sour cream has been soured with the aid of special bacteria and is usually based on single cream. *Crème fraîche* is fresh single cream treated with a culture to give a slight acidity. *Smetana* is single cream plus skimmed milk which has been carefully soured.

Buttermilk is the liquid cream left over after the cream has been used to make butter.

Yoghurt

Yoghurt is made from a mixture of whole milk, skimmed milk powder and sugars. 'Fat-free' yoghurt is made with skimmed milk. Low-fat and fat-free yoghurts will have a slightly higher carbohydrate and protein content compared with ordinary whole-milk yoghurt.

Fruit yoghurts often have additional sweetening quite apart from the sugars naturally occurring in the fruits.

A Greek-style yoghurt contains much more fat than other types – up to 5 or 6 times more.

Fromage frais is a low-fat cream cheese made from curd; its fat content depends on whether it has been made from whole or skimmed milk.

Cheese

Cheese can be *hard* such as Cheddar and Parmesan, *soft* such as Brie and Camembert, and *cottage*. The critical difference from a nutritional point of view is the amount of water they contain. Hard cheeses contain the least water, cottage cheeses the most. In terms of calories, the hard cheeses come out at *rather over* 400 kcal/100 g, the soft cheeses at about 300 and the cottage cheeses at under 100 kcal/100 g.

As you might expect, a 'full-fat' soft cheese has a high proportion of fat. In a 'cream cheese' the fat content is almost 50 per cent.

Few cheeses have significant amounts of carbohydrate.

Eggs

The calorific value of 100 g of whole raw egg is between 145 and 165 kcal. By weight 75 per cent is water, protein accounts for 12 per cent and fat 11 per cent. There is no carbohydrate to speak of. If you are counting calories it is always better to boil or poach eggs rather than frying or scrambling them in butter or oil.

Food Category or Brand	Calories /100g	Portion	Size /g	Calories /port
Generic Milks				
breastmilk, early (colostrum)	68			
breastmilk, late	78			
buttermilk, fluid	39	pint	284	110
coconut milk	53			
condensed	329			
condensed, unsweetened	154			
Crazy Milk, chocolate	63			
Crazy Milk, fruit	50			
dried, skimmed, powder	326			
dried, whole, powder	530			
evaporated	161			
Five Pints, reconstituted	46			
goat's	67			
long life, skimmed	34			
Marvel, dry	100			
Ostermilk, dry	453			
pasteurized whole	66			
semi-skimmed	46			
skimmed	35			
soya milk, sweetened	55			
soya milk, unsweetened	46			
spray-dried skimmed	51			
whole	70			
Generic Creams				
aerosol cream	343			
brandy cream	436	carton	112	488
brandy cream, thick	440	carton	112	493
cherry brandy	425	1/4 pint	112	476
clotted cream	579	1/4 pint	112	648
double cream	461	1/4 pint	112	516
double, with Cointreau	437	1/4 pint	112	489
double, fresh	462	1/4 pint	112	517
half cream	135	1/4 pint	112	151
single cream	193	1/4 pint	112	216

Food Category or Brand	Calories /100g	Portion	Size /g	Calories /port
single, fresh	219	¼ pint	112	245
Smetana, regular	129	pint	284	365
soured cream	205	¼ pint	112	230
whipping cream	321	¼ pint	112	360

Generic Yoghurts

diet types	52	carton	150	78
Greek	130	carton	150	195
low-fat, fruit	103	carton	150	155
low-fat, natural	60	carton	150	90
whole milk	62	carton	150	93

Branded Yoghurts
Asda

Greek style natural	129
Greek style with honey	150
Greek style with strawberries	127
Greek style with toffee	184
low fat apricot & mango	95
low fat banana	99
low fat black cherry	95
low fat raspberry	95
low fat rhubarb	95
low fat strawberry	91
low fat toffee	116
smooth set forest fruits	100
smooth set lemon	100
smooth set raspberry	100
smooth set strawberry	100
smooth set vanilla	100

Boots Shapers

apricot custard	56	carton		82
black cherry	57	carton		71
blackberry apple	87	carton		107
gooseberry custard	51	carton		75

Food Category or Brand	Calories /100g	Portion	Size /g	Calories /port
lemon lime yoghurts				
mousse	99	carton		89
strawberry custard	56	carton		83
strawberry yoghurt mousse	97	carton		88
strawberry	54	carton		67
toffee	55	carton		67
vanilla	53	carton		66

Chambourcy

LE YOGHURT

apricot & grapefruit		carton	125	105
pineapple & orange		carton	125	105
raspberry & lemon		carton	125	105

Dairy Crest

VERY LOW FAT

black cherry		carton	125	85
natural		carton	125	50
peach Melba		carton	125	90
raspberry		carton	125	90
strawberry		carton	125	90

THICK 'N' CREAMY

exotic fruit		carton	150	175
rhubarb		carton	150	170
strawberry & vanilla		carton	150	170

Loseley

apple		carton	150	145
apricot		carton	150	130
banana		carton	150	135
blackcurrant		carton	150	150
caramel		carton	150	170
hazelnut		carton	150	175
lemon		carton	150	150

Food Category or Brand	Calories /100g	Portion	Size /g	Calories /port
mandarin		carton	150	140
natural		carton	150	100
pineapple		carton	150	145
raisin with rum		carton	150	155
strawberry		carton	150	130

Müller

MÜLLER CRUNCH CORNER

strawberry	145	pot	150	218
toffee	161	pot	150	242
vanilla	145	pot	150	218

MÜLLER BIO CORNER

| cereal, nuts & raisins | 134 | pot | 150 | 201 |
| crunchy honey cereal | 130 | pot | 150 | 195 |

MÜLLER RICE

apple with syrup	112	pot	200	224
caramel sauce	105	pot	200	210
raisins, nutmeg with syrup	122	pot	200	244
raspberries with syrup	114	pot	200	228
strawberry with syrup	115	pot	200	230

MÜLLER LIGHT

cherry	51	pot	200	102
peach & maracuya	48	pot	200	96
pineapple & peach	49	pot	200	98
strawberry	49	pot	200	98
vanilla	50	pot	200	100

MÜLLER FRUIT CORNER

blueberry	112	pot	175	196
cherry	110	pot	175	193
peach & apricot	110	pot	175	193
pineapple & maracuya	107	pot	175	187
strawberry	118	pot	175	207

Food Category or Brand	Calories /100g	Portion	Size /g	Calories /port
Safeway				
BIO FRUIT				
apple & blackberry		pot	125	109
raspberry & redcurrant		pot	125	116
strawberry		pot	125	118
strawberry & rhubarb		pot	125	108
RICH & CREAMY				
apricot & mango		pot	150	116
peach & vanilla		pot	150	117
raspberry & redcurrant		pot	150	117
strawberry		pot	150	118
CUSTARD YOGHURT				
apricot & nectarine		pot	125	131
blackberry & apple		pot	125	131
rhubarb		pot	125	136
strawberry		pot	125	132
FRUIT TREATS				
forest fruits		pot	175	99
peach & apricot		pot	175	102
red cherry		pot	175	101
strawberry		pot	175	108
DOUBLE TREAT THICK & CREAMY				
blackcurrant & raspberry		pot	175	107
cherry		pot	175	109
peach & apricot		pot	175	107
strawberry		pot	175	106
LOW FAT				
apricot & peach		pot	150	90
cherry		pot	150	96
peach & raspberry		pot	150	98
raspberry		pot	150	91
rhubarb		pot	150	86
strawberry		pot	150	91

Food Category or Brand	Calories /100g	Portion	Size /g	Calories /port
BIO FRUIT HEALTH CHOICE				
blueberry & raspberry		pot	125	53
pineapple & mango		pot	125	51
red cherry		pot	125	54
strawberry		pot	125	53
Sainsbury's				
bio yoghurt (all flavours)		pot	125	135
economy strawberry		carton	125	108
DIET DUET				
raspberry	218	pot		87
strawberry	203	pot		82
LOW FAT				
raspberry		pot	150	152
strawberry		pot	150	122
St Michael (Marks & Spencer)				
banana smoothy			150	115
black cherry			150	110
blueberry			150	100
mango smoothy			150	110
raspberry			150	95
rhubarb			150	110
strawberry			150	100
Summer Fruit			150	100
toffee			150	120
FAT FREE				
rhubarb		each	200	105
raspberry		each	200	95

Food Category or Brand	Calories /100g	Portion	Size /g	Calories /port

Ski

SKI LOW FAT

Food	Portion	Size	Calories
apple & blackberry	carton	125	115
apple & pear	carton	125	115
apricot & mango	carton	125	127
black cherry	carton	125	130
hazelnut	carton	125	153
lemon	carton	125	118
orange & guava	carton	125	128
orange & lemon	carton	125	118
peach & passion fruit	carton	125	129
peach	carton	125	127
pineapple & grapefruit	carton	125	118
pineapple & papaya	carton	125	127
pink grapefruit	carton	125	118
plum	carton	125	115
raspberry	carton	125	126
rhubarb	carton	125	115
strawberry & cream	carton	125	124
strawberry & vanilla	carton	125	124
strawberry	carton	125	124
toffee	carton	125	160

SKI SMOOTH

Food	Portion	Size	Calories
banana	carton	125	128
blackcurrant	carton	125	127
custard	carton	125	128
peach	carton	125	127
raspberry	carton	125	127
strawberry	carton	125	127
toffee	carton	125	128
vanilla	carton	125	128

SKI LIGHT

Food	Portion	Size	Calories
blackberry & raspberry	carton	125	67
peach & pineapple	carton	125	70
red cherry	carton	125	64

Food Category or Brand	Calories /100g	Portion	Size /g	Calories /port
strawberry		carton	125	61
toffee		carton	125	60
vanilla		carton	125	58
SKI SPLITS				
forest fruits		carton	175	155
peach & pineapple		carton	175	155
red cherry		carton	175	155
strawberry		carton	175	155
SKI DEEP FILL FRUIT				
apple & blackberry		carton	175	141
peach		carton	175	141
pineapple		carton	175	141
red cherry		carton	175	141
strawberry		carton	175	141
EDEN VALE NATURAL				
natural		carton	150	102
MUNCH BUNCH YOGHURT				
apricot		carton	100	101
raspberry		carton	100	105
strawberry		carton	100	105
MUNCH BUNCH MIX-UPS				
raspberry		carton	125	150
strawberry		carton	125	152

Total

original	550			
sheep's	386			
total light	335			

Waitrose

apple & blackcurrant	97			
low fat hazelnut	112			
low fat peach melba	97			
low fat strawberry	94			
low fat toffee	165			

Food Category or Brand	Calories /100g	Portion	Size /g	Calories /port
natural bio	50			
peach & redcurrant	92			
rhubarb virtually fat free	48			
strawberry virtually fat free	50			

Branded Fromage Frais
Chambourcy

fruit, creamy	120	carton	100	120
fruit, very low fat	85	carton	100	85
natural, creamy	110	carton	100	110
natural, very low fat	50	carton	100	50

Generic and Regional Cheeses

Appenzell	403	wedge	50	202
Austrian smoked	278	wedge	50	139
Babybel	343			
Bavarian Brie, mushrooms	393	wedge	50	197
Bavarian Brie, peppers	365	wedge	50	183
Bavarian, smoked	318	wedge	50	159
Beaufort	461	wedge	50	231
Beaumont	403	wedge	50	202
Bel Paese	343	wedge	50	172
Bleu d'Auvergne	346	wedge	50	173
Bleu de Gex	414	wedge	50	207
Bleu de Velloy	403	wedge	50	202
Bleu des Causses	382	wedge	50	191
Blue	366	wedge	50	183
Blue Brie	435	wedge	50	217
Boursin	404	wedge	50	202
Bressot	262	wedge	50	131
Brie	304	wedge	50	152
Caboc	554	wedge	50	277
Caerphilly	370	wedge	50	185
Cambozola	436	wedge	50	218
Camembert	309	wedge	50	155
Cantal	496	wedge	50	248

Food Category or Brand	Calories /100g	Portion	Size /g	Calories /port
Chaumes	375	wedge	50	188
Cheddar	425	wedge	50	213
Cheshire	389	wedge	50	195
Cheviot	414	wedge	50	207
Chevret	303	wedge	50	152
cottage, uncreamed	388	portion	50	194
cream	813	portion	50	407
cream cheese, chives	439	wedge	50	220
cream cheese, natural	439	wedge	50	220
cream cheese, pineapple	386	wedge	50	193
curd	123	wedge	50	62
Danbo	346	wedge	50	173
Danish Blue	366	wedge	50	183
Danish Elbo	346	wedge	50	173
Danish Esrom	336	wedge	50	168
Danish Fynbo	361	wedge	50	181
Danish Havarti	439	wedge	50	220
Danish Maribo	368	wedge	50	184
Danish Mellow Blue	400	wedge	50	200
Danish Mycella	364	wedge	50	182
Danish Saga	461	wedge	50	231
Danish Samsoe	368	wedge	50	184
Danish Svenbo	382	wedge	50	191
Danish Tybo	325	wedge	50	163
Derby	403	wedge	50	202
Dolcellata	357	wedge	50	179
Double Gloucester	388	wedge	50	194
Edam	313	wedge	50	157
Edelweiss	393	wedge	50	197
Emmenthal	370	wedge	50	185
Etorki	478	wedge	50	239
Feta, Danish cow's	261	wedge	50	131
Feta, Greek ewe's	303	wedge	50	152
fondue mix	264			
full fat soft cheese, garlic, parsley	307	wedge	50	154

Food Category or Brand	Calories /100g	Portion	Size /g	Calories /port
Gaperon	303	wedge	50	152
German smoked	346	wedge	50	173
Gjetost	478	wedge	50	239
Gorgonzola	393	wedge	50	197
Gouda	340	wedge	50	170
Gouda, matured	390	wedge	50	195
Graindorge Livarot	328	wedge	50	164
Gruyère	465	wedge	50	233
Halali Limburger	261	wedge	50	131
Halumi	300	wedge	50	150
Jarlsberg	350	wedge	50	175
Lancashire	350	wedge	50	175
Langres	396	wedge	50	198
Leiden	407	wedge	50	204
Maasdam	475	wedge	50	238
Manchego	489	wedge	50	245
Mariolles	378	wedge	50	189
Mascapone	400	wedge	50	200
Melbury	325	wedge	50	163
Momolette	318	wedge	50	159
Morbier	375	wedge	50	188
Mozarella	279	wedge	50	139
Munster	328	wedge	50	164
Niolo	400	wedge	50	200
Norwegian Blue	357	wedge	50	179
Olivet	343	wedge	50	172
Orangerulle	328	wedge	50	164
Orkney	411	wedge	50	206
Orkney Claymore	396	wedge	50	198
Parmesan	420	sprinkling	5	21
Picodon	257	wedge	50	129
Port Salut	315	wedge	50	158
Primat des Gaulles	482	wedge	50	241
processed	374	wedge	50	187
Pyramide	350	wedge	50	175
Quark	88	wedge	50	44

Food Category or Brand	Calories /100g	Portion	Size /g	Calories /port
Rambol with walnuts	418	wedge	50	209
Red Leicester	396	wedge	50	198
Red Windsor	407	wedge	50	204
Ricotta	146	wedge	50	73
Rigotte	350	wedge	50	175
Rollot	432	wedge	50	216
Roquefort	378	wedge	50	189
roule, garlic & herbs	329	wedge	50	165
roule, light	179	wedge	50	90
roule, spices	318	wedge	50	159
Royalp	393	wedge	50	197
Sage Derby	407	wedge	50	204
Sardo Pecorino	453	wedge	50	227
Shropshire blue	414	wedge	50	207
skimmed milk	82	wedge	50	41
smoked	390	wedge	50	195
Somerset goat's, natural	314	wedge	50	157
soya cheese	321	wedge	50	161
spread	290	spread	10	29
Sprinz	443	wedge	50	222
St Albray	343	wedge	50	172
St Ivel	380	wedge	50	190
St Nectaire	353	wedge	50	177
St Pauline	300	wedge	50	150
St Pecorino	453	wedge	50	227
Stilton, blue	418	wedge	50	209
Stilton, white	368	wedge	50	184
Taleggio	361	wedge	50	181
Tartare	443	wedge	50	222
Tartare, light	156	wedge	50	168
Tilsiter	418	wedge	50	209
Tomme blanche	400	wedge	50	200
Tomme grasse tourre	375	wedge	50	188
Torta	389	wedge	50	195
Vacherin Mont d'Or	339	wedge	50	170
Welsh goat's, herbs	307	wedge	50	154

Food Category or Brand	Calories /100g	Portion	Size /g	Calories /port
Welsh goat's, natural	307	wedge	50	154
Welsh goat's, peppers	307	wedge	50	154
Wensleydale	406	wedge	50	203
Yarg	386	wedge	50	193

Generic Cottage Cheese

natural	102	1 carton	113	115
Cheddar-type	117	1 carton	227	265
Cheddar & onion	119	1 carton	113	135
chicken & mushroom	124	1 carton	113	140
fruit	117	1 carton	227	265
half-fat	84	1 carton	113	95
Mexican chicken	102	1 carton	113	115
onion & chive	95	1 carton	227	215
pineapple	97	1 carton	113	110
prawns	146	1 carton	113	165
salmon & cucumber	128	1 carton	113	145
spring onion	96	1 carton	225	215

Branded Cottage Cheeses

St Ivel Shape

cheese, onion & chive	90
cherry tomato & basil	73
pineapple	82
plain	72

Primula

cheese spread, original	257
cheese spread, chives	253
cheese spread, ham	253
cheese spread, shrimp	253

Generic Eggs

duck's	190	1 egg		115
hen's, dried	580			

Food Category or Brand	Calories /100g	Portion	Size /g	Calories /port
hen's, fresh, whole	163	1 egg		80
hen's, fried	239	1 egg		70
hen's, in an omelette	172	1 egg		55
hen's, poached	160	1 egg		50
hen's, scrambled	172	1 egg		55
hen's, white	37	1 white		15
hen's, yolk	350	1 yolk		60
quail's	99	1 egg		15

Desserts

Most desserts are treats rather than contributions to a low-calorie diet. A range has been included so that you can see just how damaging they can be. For the slimmer, the ideal dessert is fresh, unsweetened fruit, or some low-fat, unsweetened dairy products (see the sections on **Fruit** and **Dairy Products**). Thereafter, almost everything is bad news: even plain stewed fruit is nearly always sweetened with sugar in various forms. Beyond that you are eating considerable amounts of pastry (flour, butter, eggs), other forms of complex carbohydrate, and cream and other high-fat dairy products.

There are separate sections on Cakes and Biscuits and Ice-cream.

Food Category or Brand	Calories /100g	Portion	Size /g	Calories /port
Generic Desserts				
apple dumpling	202	1 portion	135	270
apple pudding	239	1 portion	135	320
apple pie	190	1 portion	135	255
banana custard	103	1 portion	135	140

Food Category or Brand	Calories /100g	Portion	Size /g	Calories /port
blancmange	118	1 portion	135	150
bread & butter pudding	162	1 portion	135	220
canary pudding	462	1 portion	135	620
castle pudding, steamed	396	1 portion	135	530
chocolate mould	125	1 portion	135	170
custard powder (prepared)	116			
custard tart	290	1 portion	135	390
dumplings	206	1 portion	135	275
egg custard, baked	113			
egg custard, sauce	119			
gooseberry pie	180	1 portion	135	240
jam omelette	276	1 portion	100	275
jam roll, baked	403	1 portion	135	540
jelly, milk	111	1 portion	135	150
Leicester pudding	685	1 portion	135	925
meringue	393	1 portion	135	530
mixed fruit	325	1 portion	135	435
pancakes	301	1 portion	75	225
plum pie	183	1 portion	135	245
queen of puddings	213	1 portion	135	285
rhubarb pie	188	1 portion	135	250
rice pudding	144	1 portion	135	195
sago pudding	127	1 portion	135	170
semolina pudding	131	1 portion	135	175
suet pudding, plain	370	1 portion	135	495
suet pudding, with raisins	352	1 portion	135	470
syrup pudding	368	1 portion	135	490
tapioca pudding	129	1 portion	135	175
treacle tart	375	1 portion	135	500
trifle	150	1 portion	135	200

Food Category or Brand	Calories /100g	Portion	Size /g	Calories /port
Branded Desserts				
Ambrosia				
chocolate rice	100	1 can	425	425
creamed rice	91	1 can	425	387
creamed rice with sultanas				
& nutmeg	101	1 can	425	429
creamed sago	80	1 can	425	340
Devon custard	101	1 can	425	429
low-fat Devon custard	73	1 can	425	310
Asda				
bread and butter pudding	248			
chocolate mousse	184			
creme caramel	102			
fresh cream fruit trifle	202			
jam roly poly with custard	235			
sherry trifle	172			
spotted dick with custard	222			
sticky toffee pudding	319			
strawberry cheesecake	218			
toffee cheesecake	188			
FROZEN				
American chocolate				
cheesecake	393			
apple and blackberry pie	279			
apple crumble	193			
Black Forest gateau	238			
cherry cheesecake	184			
chocolate eclairs	359			
chocolate pudding	319			
raspberry pavlova	300			
toffee pavlova	368			

Food Category or Brand	Calories /100g	Portion	Size /g	Calories /port
Birds				
ANGEL DELIGHT				
banana	490			
butterscotch	475			
chocolate	455			
forest fruit	490			
raspberry	490			
strawberry	485			
toffee	480			
vanilla ice cream	490			
ANGEL DELIGHT, SUGAR FREE				
banana toffee	495			
butterscotch	480			
chocolate	450			
raspberry	465			
strawberry	495			
tangerine	495			
vanilla ice cream	500			
Boots				
Just lemon	28	1 carton		39
Just fruit	43	1 carton		61
Strawberry delight	79	1 carton		96
Chambourcy				
Black Forest dessert		1 carton		140
cherry cheesecake		1 carton		215
chocolate crème Vienna		1 carton		150
pot au crème		1 carton		145
real chocolate mousse		1 carton		120
real crème caramel		1 carton		110
real fruit mousse		1 carton		105
strawberry cheesecake		1 carton		215

Food Category or Brand	Calories /100g	Portion	Size /g	Calories /port
LE DESSERT CUP				
almond toffee		1 carton		155
chocolate coconut		1 carton		155
chocolate orange		1 carton		205
LE GRAND				
chocolate & vanilla		1 carton		270
strawberry & vanilla		1 carton		260

Chivers

table jellies, all flavours	290			
FRUIT FOR ALL				
apricot	115			
blackcurrant	110			
morello cherry	110			
JELLY CREAMS				
chocolate	365			
other flavours	370			

Edenvale

banana supreme	105			
blackcurrant cheesecake	207			
Black Forest trifle	152			
caramel supreme	127			
chocolate supreme	134			
chocomousse	180			
crème caramel	139			
crème orange	141			
crème raspberry	141			
fruit softy	129			
pear Hélène sundae	132			
raspberry cheesecake	194			

Food Category or Brand	Calories /100g	Portion	Size /g	Calories /port
raspberry trifle	153			
Spanish orange trifle	155			
strawberry cheesecake	196			
strawberry trifle	160			
tropical supreme	116			

Heinz (tinned)

Food Category or Brand	Calories /100g	Portion	Size /g	Calories /port
chocolate sponge, chocolate sauce	219			
mixed fruit sponge	226			
strawberry jam sponge	220			
treacle sponge	211			
Weight Watchers rice pudding	72	1 can	425	305

Lyons

Food Category or Brand	Calories /100g	Portion	Size /g	Calories /port
apple dessert pie		1 packet		1160
chocolate sponge pudding		1 packet		190
jam sponge pudding		1 packet		210
lemon meringue pie		1 packet		1415

McVitie's

Food Category or Brand	Calories /100g	Portion	Size /g	Calories /port
apple crumble	254			
apple dumplings	261			
apple pie	239			
chocolate & orange royale	289			
Chocolova	375			
Dutch apple tart	236			
jam roly poly	400			
nut meringue gateau	407			
profiteroles	475			
queen of puddings	207			
raspberry torte	275			
spotted dick	361			
strawberry pavlova	336			
tiramisu	329			

Food Category or Brand	Calories /100g	Portion	Size /g	Calories /port
CHEESECAKES				
blackcurrant	396			
cherry	339			
chocolate truffle	386			
St Clements deep & creamy	343			
Mr Kipling (Frozen)				
apple & blackcurrant crumble	264			
apple crumble	246			
golden syrup sponge	361			
rich jam roly poly	207			
spotted dick	354			
Müller				
low-fat rice desserts	70			
Nestlé				
custard powder, dry	330			
Double Top topping	178			
Tip Top topping	110			
Ross				
jam roly poly	381	1 packet	250	953
spotted dick	429	1 packet	275	1180
Rowntree				
jelly, all flavours	268			
instant custard mix, dry	416			
Safeway				
blackcurrant cheesecake		each	90	272
cherry trifle		each	113	189
choc trifle		each	113	255
chocolate cheesecake		each	92	302
chocolate mousse		each	62.5	205

Food Category or Brand	Calories /100g	Portion	Size /g	Calories /port
chocolate peanut clusters		each	140	156
chocolate surprise dessert		each	150	189
creme caramel		each	128	103
fruit cocktail		each	113	182
gooseberry fruit fool		each	114	201
Italian mandolato		each	113	269
milk & white chocolate crispies		each	140	161
raspberry fruit fool		each	140	124
real fruit fool		each	114	174
savers choc mousse		each	60	173
strawberry cheesecake		each	90	262
tiramisu		each	100	265
toffee surprise dessert		each	150	195

Sainsbury's

Food Category or Brand	Calories /100g	Portion	Size /g	Calories /port
blackcurrant trifle		carton		196
caramel surprise		carton		185
chocolate trifle		carton		271
creamed rice		can		396
crème caramel		carton		102
economy rice pudding		can		340
fruit cocktail trifle		carton		209
gooseberry fool		carton		212
Italian tartuffo		pot		269
lemon baverois		pot		175
low fat apricot fool		carton		90
low fat choc mousse		carton		75
low fat gooseberry fool		pot		81
low fat rice pudding		can		366
rhubarb fool		carton		151
strawberry fool		carton		189
strawberry trifle		carton		194

Food Category or Brand	Calories /100g	Portion Size /g	Calories /port
FROZEN DESSERTS			
apple strudel	299		
Black Forest gateau	310		
blackcurrant cheesecake	255		
choc fudge cheesecake	362		
lemon torte	240		
raspberry pavlova	273		
strawberry gateau	263		
summer fruit brulee	296		
tiramisu	336		
woodland fruit strudel	289		
St Michael (Marks & Spencer)			
American chocolate brownie	245		
apple pie	250		
Bakewell tart	460		
chocolate cheesecake	380		
fruit trifle	205		
jam roly poly	240		
jam sponge	311		
lemon cheesecake	350		
lemon meringue pie	360		
lemon tart	415		
Manchester tart	370		
panacotta	285		
passion fruit brulee	265		
spotted dick	302		
sticky toffee pudding	275		
tarte citron	350		
tiramisu	290		
toffee pecan tart	455		
treacle tart	380		

Food Category or Brand	Calories /100g	Portion	Size /g	Calories /port
FROZEN				
bramley apple pie	260			
chocolate cheesecake	376			
chocolate eclairs	345			
chocolate layer gateau	323			
lemon meringue pie	261			
lemon tortes	270			
lemon/lime gateau	295			
raspberry brulee cheesecake	264			
raspberry pavlova	230			
raspberry roulade	315			
toffee pecan pavlova	420			
toffee roulade	423			
Sara Lee				
raspberry fromage dessert		1 packet		810

Drinks

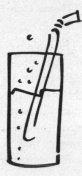

Alcoholic Drinks

The energy in alcoholic drinks comes partly from the alcohol and partly from sugars. One gram of pure alcohol provides the body with 7 kcal of energy.

An ordinary beer contains between 3 and 6 g of alcohol per 100 ml of fluid. (A half-pint is 280 ml, a common can size is 330 ml).

An ordinary cider contains just under 4 g of alcohol per 100 ml, but vintage cider might be over 10 g of alcohol per 100 ml.

For convenience the low- and no-alcohol versions are also included here rather than with the soft drinks that are listed in the 'non-alcoholic drinks' table. A no-alcohol beer will obviously have no calories from alcohol but is still likely to contain sugars.

Wines have between 8 and 10 g of alcohol per 100 ml.

Fortified wines – port, sherry and so on – are around 15 to 16 g of alcohol per 100 ml and 40-per-cent-volume spirits (the usual strength) are about 32 g of alcohol per 100 ml. Port may be up to 12 per cent carbohydrate (in the form of sugars) but some liqueurs, for example cherry brandy, may be over 30 per cent sugar.

The table below shows the relationship between an alcohol's strength – shown as percentage volume – and the weight of alcohol per 100 g of liquid. The figure on the far right is the calorific content of the alcohol; many of these drinks will have a higher actual calorific content, however, because of the additional sugars – a medium sherry, for example, may have 3.5 g of carbohydrate, pushing the calorific value per 100 g from 99.9 to 118.

Alcohol – Relationship between Percentage Volume and Calories

Drink	% vol	alcohol g /100g	cal /100ml
spirits	40	31.7	222.0
spirits	37.5	29.7	208.1
sloe gin	25	19.8	138.8
peach schnapps	23	18.2	127.6
freezomint	20	15.9	111.0
sherry	18	14.3	99.9
Bailey's	17	13.5	94.3
Taboo	14.9	11.8	82.7
Dubonnet	14.7	11.6	81.6
Sanatogen	14.5	11.5	80.5

Hot Drinks

By themselves, neither tea nor coffee have any calorific value – any sugar or milk added does. Each teaspoon of sugar is 20 calories. A dash of milk – say 30 ml – is another 20 calories. Most herbal teas similarly have no calorific value, but those infusions based on fruits may have inherent sugars.

Cocoa and chocolate-based drinks, and those with malt in them, may be based either on powdered whole milk or on semi-skimmed or skimmed milk. While some chocolate drinks simply require the addition of water, most of the older varieties expect you to add milk.

There is a separate Soups listing; however, at the end of the Hot Drinks table there is a section on the drinks and convenience soups sold from vending machines.

Non-Alcoholic Drinks

Nearly all commercially manufactured non-alcoholic drinks contain large amounts of added sugar or sweeteners. Fruits themselves are chiefly glucose and fructose, but apples and pears also include sucrose.

The packaging on fruit juices needs to be read with particular care: only the most expensive brands are solely 'juice' in the sense that you end up with the drink you would make at home by squeezing a piece of fresh fruit. Usually the flesh – and sometimes part of the skin – is pulped and heat-treated.

The fruits used in juices made 'from concentrate' are kept in concentrated form and then diluted when placed in the carton or bottle which you eventually buy.

Squashes are drink concentrates; you must divide the figures supplied in the table by the amount you dilute them.

Carbonation – injecting bubbles to produce a fizzy drink – has no direct effect on calorific value, but the process usually adds an acidic taste which the manufacturer then counteracts by adding sugars.

'Diet' and 'Lo-Cal' drinks use artificial sweeteners.

Glucose drinks such as Lucozade are made from glucose syrup and thus have very high calorific values – fine if you are an athlete or invalid, bad news if you are slimming.

This section also includes milk shakes, as opposed to flavoured milks, which are located in the **Dairy Products** section.

You will also find some soft drinks and milk shakes in the **Fast Foods** section.

Food Category or Brand	Calories /100ml	Portion	Size /ml	Calories /port
Branded Beers				
Bass				
draught	36	1 can	440	160
Beamish				
canned	34	1 can	440	150
draught	32	1/2 pint	284	90
Bentley				
bottles	28	1 bottle	284	80
Burton's				
canned	41	1 can	440	180
draught	42	1/2 pint	284	120
Courage				
draught	35	1/2 pint	284	100
Double Diamond				
canned	38	1 can	440	165
draught	32	1/2 pint	284	90
Ind Coope				
bottled	27	1 bottle	275	75
draught	28	1/2 pint	284	80
John Bull				
draught	30	1/2 pint	284	85

Food Category or Brand	Calories /100ml	Portion	Size /ml	Calories /port
John Smith's				
canned	36	1 can	440	160
draught	33	½ pint	284	95
London Pride				
draught	37	½ pint	284	105
McEwans Export				
canned	36	1 can	440	160
Newcastle Brown				
bottled	38	1 bottle	440	165
Ruddles				
draught	35	½ pint	284	100
Stones				
draught	32	½ pint	284	90
Tartan				
canned	31	1 can	440	138
Tetley				
canned	32	1 can	440	140
Walkers				
draught	28	½ pint	284	80
Watney's				
draught	33	½ pint	284	95
Webster's				
draught	32	½ pint	284	90

Food Category or Brand	Calories /100ml	Portion	Size /ml	Calories /port
Worthington's				
canned	27	1 can	440	120

Low- and No-alcohol Branded Beers
LA Bitter

bottled	24	1 bottle	275	65
John Smith's				
bottled	16	1 bottle	275	45
McEwan's LA				
canned	15	1 can	440	65
Swan Light				
canned	17	1 can	440	75
White Label				
canned	31	1 can	440	135

Branded Lagers
Budweiser

draught	39	½ pint	284	110
Carling Black Label				
canned	32	1 can	440	140
Carlsberg				
bottled	45	1 bottle	275	125
Castlemaine XXXX				
canned	38	1 can	440	165

Food Category or Brand	Calories /100ml	Portion	Size /ml	Calories /port
Foster's				
canned	40	1 can	375	150
draught	32	½ pint	284	90
Heineken				
bottled	31	1 bottle	275	85
Hofmeister				
canned	30	1 can	440	130
draught	30	½ pint	284	85
Holsten Export				
draught	40	½ pint	284	115
Holsten Pils				
canned	39	1 can	440	170
Kestrel				
canned	26	1 can	440	115
Kronenbourg				
canned	42	1 can	440	185
draught	42	½ pint	284	120
Lamot Pils				
canned	38	1 can	440	165
Löwenbräu Pils				
canned	41	1 can	440	180
Skol				
canned	28	1 can	440	125

Food Category or Brand	Calories /100ml	Portion	Size /ml	Calories /port
Stella Artois				
canned	42	1 can	440	185
Tennent's				
canned	32	1 can	440	140
draught	33	1/2 pint	284	95

Extra-strength Branded Lagers

Carlsberg Special Brew				
bottled	75	1 bottle	275	205
Kestrel Super Strength				
canned	75	1 can	440	330
Skol Extra Strength				
canned	70	1 can	440	310
Tennents Super				
canned	73	1 can	440	320

Low- and No-alcohol Branded Lagers

Barbican				
bottled	12	1 bottle	275	35
Carlton				
draught	18	1/2 pint	284	50
Miller Lite				
canned	27	1 can	440	120
draught	26	1/2 pint	284	75
Swan				
canned	19	1 can	375	70

Food Category or Brand	Calories /100ml	Portion	Size /ml	Calories /port
Tennent's LA				
canned	18	1 can	440	80
Branded Ciders				
Blackthorn				
dry, bottled	35	1 bottle	275	95
Copperhead				
canned	35	1 can	440	154
dry, draught	30	1/2 pint	284	85
dry, strong, draught	35	1 bottle	275	96
Country Manor				
medium dry, draught	55	1/2 pint	284	155
medium sweet, draught	63	1/2 pint	284	180
rosé, draught	46	1/2 pint	284	130
sparkling, draught	60	1/2 pint	284	170
Diamond White				
bottled	53	1 bottle	275	145
Merrydown				
country, draught	49	1/2 pint	284	140
traditional, draught	46	1/2 pint	284	130
vintage, draught	60	1/2 pint	284	170
vintage dry, draught	53	1/2 pint	284	150
Red Rock				
bottled	41	1 bottle	330	135
Strongbow				
draught	36	1/2 pint	284	101

Food Category or Brand	Calories /100ml	Portion	Size /ml	Calories /port
Taunton Cool				
bottled	35	1 bottle	275	95
Woodpecker				
draught	35	1/2 pint	284	100
Generic Wines				
champagne	70	glass	115	80
red, dry	70	glass	115	80
red, sweet	87	glass	115	100
rosé	74	glass	115	85
sparkling	78	glass	115	90
white, dry	65	glass	115	75
white, sweet	91	glass	115	105
Generic Fortified Wines				
ruby or tawny	150	measure	50	75
port, vintage	160	measure	50	80
port, white	100	measure	50	70
sherry, cream	126	measure	50	63
sherry, dry	100	measure	50	54
sherry, medium	116	measure	50	58
Generic Spirits				
brandy, apricot	240	measure	25	60
brandy, average	200	measure	25	50
gin	200	measure	25	50
rum	200	measure	25	50
vodka	200	measure	25	50
whisky	200	measure	25	50
Branded Spirits				
Bacardi	200	measure	25	50
Jack Daniels	240	measure	25	60

Food Category or Brand	Calories /100ml	Portion	Size /ml	Calories /port
Martini				
Bianco	134	measure	50	67
Extra Dry	134	measure	50	67
Rosso	170	measure	50	85
Pernod	244	measure	25	61
Pimms	196	measure	50	98
Southern Comfort	280	measure	25	70
Branded Liqueurs				
Advocaat	260	measure	25	65
Bailey's Irish Cream	320	measure	25	80
Benedictine	360	measure	25	90
Cassis	260	measure	25	65
Cointreau	340	measure	25	85
Drambuie	340	measure	25	85
Grand Marnier	320	measure	25	80
Irish Velvet	380	measure	25	95
Kirsch	200	measure	25	50
Mardi Gras	200	measure	25	50
Tia Maria	300	measure	25	75

Food Category or Brand	Calories /100ml	Portion	Size /ml	Calories /port
Generic Hot Drinks				
tea, Indian	1			
coffee	2			
Branded Hot Drinks				
Bovril		1 tsp		10
Cadbury's				
Bournvita		1tsp		22
Bournvita Break		1 sachet		110
Drinking Chocolate		2 tsps		40
Highlights		sachet		40
Horlicks				
low-fat		sachet		129
low-fat chocolate		sachet		124
Marvel		1 tsp		6
Milk Chocolate Break		1 sachet		105
Plain Chocolate Break		1 sachet		105
Carnation				
Build Up		1 sachet		130
Slim Chocolate		1 sachet		41
Tea-mate		1 tsp		10
Horlicks				
Instant		1 sachet		105
Instant Chocolate Malted		1 sachet		125
Instant Hot Chocolate		1 sachet		130
Lift				
lemon tea		2 tsps		35
London Herb & Spice Co.				
Natural Break		1 cup		5

Food Category or Brand	Calories /100ml	Portion	Size /ml	Calories /port
Nestlé				
cappuccino, original		cup		48
cappuccino, unsweetened		cup		47
Elevenses		1 tsp		5
Milo		1 tsp		24
Novartis Nutrition UK Ltd				
instant ovaltine light		1 sachet		75
(using hot water)		3/4 tsp (jar)		75
ovaltine power		1 sachet		92
(using hot water)		2 level scoops (jar)		92
traditional ovaltine		3/4 heaped tsp		192
(using semi-skimmed milk)				
Options				
choc & ginger		1 sachet		38
choc & Irish cream		1 sachet		37
choc & mint		1 sachet		38
choc & mocha		1 sachet		36
choc & orange		1 sachet		39
choc & toffee		1 sachet		38
choc & Turkish delight		1 sachet		38
choc au lait		1 sachet		39
hot toffee		1 sachet		54
white chocolate		1 sachet		55
(all using hot water)				
Options Midnight (using hot water)				
choc & brandy		1 sachet		38
choc & coffee liqueur		1 sachet		38
choc & orange liqueur		1 sachet		38
choc & rum and raisin		1 sachet		38

Food Category or Brand	Calories /100ml	Portion	Size /ml	Calories /port
Oxo				
beef drink		1 tsp		5
cubes, all flavours		1 cube		15
Sainsbury's				
cappuccino		sachet		46
duos, hot instant choc		sachet		38
instant hot choc		serving		122
Superdrug				
Supatrim instant chocolate		1 sachet		40
Supatrim malted milk		1 sachet		40
Symingtons				
dandelion coffee		1 tsp		15
Typhoo				
QT instant white tea		cup		11
Generic Fruit Juices				
blood orange	39	1/4 pint	142	55
clementine	49	1/4 pint	142	70
grapefruit	39	1/4 pint	142	55
minneola	39	1/4 pint	142	55
orange	32	1/4 pint	142	45
orange & grapefruit	32	1/4 pint	142	45
ortanique	39	1/4 pint	142	55
pineapple	42	1/4 pint	142	60
pineapple & grapefruit	49	1/4 pint	142	70
pink grapefruit	42	1/4 pint	142	60

Food Category or Brand	Calories /100ml	Portion	Size /ml	Calories /port
Branded Fruit and Vegetable Juices				
Asda				
cranberry/raspberry	54			
peach Melba	45			
pure apple	47			
pure orange and pineapple	46			
pure orange	45			
pure pineapple	47			
Boots Shapers				
tropical	49	250ml		128
unsweetened orange	42	250ml		110
Libby's				
apple 'C'	45			
blackcurrant 'C'	42			
grapefruit	38			
grapefruit 'C', sweetened	58			
orange, sweetened	51			
orange, unsweetened	33			
orange 'C', sweetened	51			
pineapple	53			
tomato	20			
umbongo fruit	41			
Lindavia				
apple, clear	42			
apple, unfiltered	45			
apricot	60			
blackberry	29			
blackcurrant	56			
carrot	23			
cherry	55			
grapefruit	22			
orange	42			

Food Category or Brand	Calories /100ml	Portion	Size /ml	Calories /port
passionfruit	34			
peach	37			
pear	45			
plum	64			
redcurrant	57			
red & white grape	63			
tomato	18			
vegetable	30			
Longlife				
apple & mango	46	¼ pint	142	65
English apple	39	¼ pint	142	55
mandarin	39	¼ pint	142	55
orange & apricot	46	¼ pint	142	65
red grapefruit	32	¼ pint	142	45
Safeway				
Florida orange & mango	42			
freshly squeezed grapefruit	36			
freshly squeezed orange	40			
pink Florida grapefruit	41			
pressed pineapple	48			
pure orange	45			
ruby red orange	55			
Sainsbury's				
freshly squeezed orange	49			
pineapple & coconut	52			
pure apple	45			
pure orange	47			
pure pineapple	53			
tropical fruit drink	52			

Food Category or Brand	Calories /100ml	Portion	Size /ml	Calories /port
St Michael (Marks & Spencer)				
apple & mango			250	235
cranberry juice			1000	60
freshly squeezed grape & raspberry			250	55
freshly squeezed grapefruit			250	30
freshly squeezed orange			250	41
pressed apple			250	52
Spar				
'8' fruit drink	44			
grapefruit	31			
orange	39			
pure apple	42			
'Saver' Breakfast Orange	41			
Waitrose				
apple	45			
apple & mango	52			
grapefruit	50			
orange	46			
pineapple	47			
tomato juice	21			
white grape	62			
Branded Carbonated Drinks				
Barr				
Iron-Bru	40	1 can	330	132
Shandy	32	1 can	330	106
Tizer	40	1 can	330	132
Vimto	26	1 can	330	86
Boots Shapers				
apple and grape	2		500	10
cloudy lemonade	3		500	13
forest fruit	1		500	5

Food Category or Brand	Calories /100ml	Portion	Size /ml	Calories /port
kiwi and lime	1		500	5
peach	1		500	5
Britvic				
ginger ale, dry	22	1 can	330	73
ginger beer	42	1 can	330	139
lime, lemon, orange	50	1 can	330	165
tonic water	31	1 can	330	102
Coca-Cola				
caffeine-free Coke	0	1 can	330	0
Coca Cola	41	1 can	330	135
Diet Coke	0	1 can	330	0
Cherry Coke	42	1 can	330	140
Corona				
cherryade	26	1 bottle	250	65
lemonade	24	1 bottle	250	60
orangeade	28	1 bottle	250	70
Fanta				
cream soda	28	1 can	330	92
ginger beer	31	1 can	330	102
lemonade	24	1 can	330	79
orangeade	33	1 can	330	109
raspberryade	29	1 can	330	96
sparkling lemon	35	1 can	330	116
Lucozade				
barley, lemon & orange	72	1 can	330	238
glucose	73	1 can	330	241
Isotonic Orange	26	1 can	330	86
Sport	11	1 can	330	36

Food Category or Brand	Calories /100ml	Portion	Size /ml	Calories /port
Sainsbury's				
classic cola		glass	250	110
diet classic cola		glass	250	1
Schweppes				
bitter lemon	33	1 can	330	109
bitter orange	44	1 can	330	145
ginger ale	22	1 can	330	73
ginger ale, dry	16	1 can	330	53
ginger beer	35	1 can	330	116
lemonade	25	1 can	330	83
lemonade shandy	26	1 can	330	86
orange	39	1 can	330	129
Russian	22	1 can	330	73
strawberry	36	1 can	330	119
tonic water	19	1 can	330	63
Tropical Spring	30	1 can	330	99
Tango				
apple	36	1 can	330	119
grapefruit	42	1 can	330	139
lemon with lime	35	1 can	330	116
orange	45	1 can	330	149
White's				
cherryade	20	1 can	330	66
cream soda	20	1 can	330	66
dandelion & burdock	25	1 can	330	83
ginger beer	29	1 can	330	96
lemonade	20	1 can	330	66
lemonade, traditional	28	1 can	330	92
orangeade	23	1 can	330	76

Food Category or Brand	Calories /100ml	Portion	Size /ml	Calories /port
Branded Squashes				
Britvic				
blackcurrant	122			
high-juice lemon	128			
high-juice lime	134			
high-juice orange	128			
lemon	96			
orange	108			
peppermint	92			
Robinson's				
lemon barley	105			
lime juice	140			
orange barley	110			
original lemon	140			
original orange	155			
Sainsbury's				
blackcurrant hi-juice		serving		105
economy orange drink		serving		6
hi-juice lemon squash		serving		94
whole lemon drink		serving		23
Waitrose				
apple & blackcurrant	8			
apple & strawberry	16			
citrus	23			
exotic fruit	41			
orange	113			
orange & mango	46			
tropical drink	15			

Food Category or Brand	Calories /100ml	Portion	Size /ml	Calories /port
Branded Milk Shakes				
Cadbury's				
chocolate milk	93	1 carton	200	185
Crusha Syrup				
banana	111			
black cherry	167			
chocolate	116			
lime	95			
pineapple	107			
raspberry	106			
strawberry	107			
vanilla	198			
Dairy Crest				
banana	60	1 carton	200	120
chocolate	63	1 carton	200	125
strawberry	60	1 carton	200	120
Edenvale				
made up, all flavours	75	glass	150	113
Mars				
milk drink	100	1 carton	200	200
Nestlé				
Nesquik with whole milk, all flavours	170	1 glass	150	
Sainsbury's				
Mr Bump banana milk shake		bottle		177
strawberry milk drink		glass	250	188

Food Category or Brand	Calories /100ml	Portion	Size /ml	Calories /port
St Michael (Marks & Spencer)				
banana milk	74			
banana milkshake			330	248
chocolate milk			250	213
chocolate milkshake			330	281
strawberry milk			250	193
strawberry milkshake			330	248
Spar				
banana	50	1 glass	150	
chocolate	60	1 glass	150	
strawberry	50	1 glass	150	

Ethnic Foods

These 'exotic' foods are the popular dishes you will find on many restaurant menus. It would have been preferable to include cuisines from rather more cultures, but nutritional data is scarce for the less common styles of cooking. Obviously each chef will make each dish slightly differently and restaurants vary considerably in the size of portions offered, so these calorific figures are 'indicative' rather than precise.

Various ethnic dishes, both chilled and frozen, are also available from supermarkets. You will find a range of these in the **Ready-made Meals** section.

You can often guess at the calorific value of an individual item if you know a little about the cooking method involved. Here are some generalizations about low-calorie choices for each form of popular cuisine:

- Chinese: avoid 'sweet-and-sour' type sauces and have plain, boiled rice rather than any other kind. Select simple stir-fried dishes, and meats that have been roasted or wind-dried.
- French: French sauces can contain large amounts of carbohydrate and fats. As a main course stick with

those made with wine rather than cream or cheese
sauces. Better still, look for simple grills. Choose clear
soups rather than thickened ones. Ask for fresh fruit
for dessert.

- Greek: Greek salads often have feta cheese; but this is
  still a better choice than taramasalata or houmous,
  which is made with olive oil. The charcoal grill is an
  important part of Greek cooking and almost anything
  from that will be relatively 'safe' – you can have fish as
  well as kebabs. Moussaka has large amounts of dairy
  product in the sauce and slimmers should avoid it.
  Almost all the Greek pastries are very fattening as they
  are drenched in honey.

- Indian: the best slimmer's choices come from the
  tandoor, the clay oven from which you get chicken
  tandoori, tikka and seekh kebab. Of the various Indian
  sauces, Madras is the most fattening. A lot of Indian
  cooking is done with *ghee* – clarified butter. The
  figures given for biriyani dishes may be misunderstood:
  a biriyani is a complete main course; the others are
  elements from which you make up your meal.

- Italian: on the whole, the Italian cuisine is not for
  those on a slimming diet. Look mostly for salads and
  simple stuffed vegetable dishes. The problem is not so
  much pizza and pasta themselves (tables for which are
  in the **Rice, Pasta and Pizza** section) but their very
  rich sauces, which often include cheese and sometimes
  egg. A carbonara sauce has the highest calorific value.

Food Category or Brand	Calories /100g	Portion	Size /g	Calories /port
Chinese				
barbecue spare ribs		each		140
beef in oyster sauce		1 portion		345
butterfly prawns, in batter		1 portion		365
chicken chop suey		1 portion		425
chicken chow mein, noodles		1 portion		715
crab & sweetcorn soup		1 portion		155
egg fu yung		1 portion		745
fried rice		1 portion		555
king prawns in batter		each		185
prawn chop suey		1 portion		310
prawn crackers		each		15
shredded beef		1 portion		540
sweet & sour pork		1 portion		860
sweet & sour prawns		1 portion		470
Desserts				
apple fritter		each		65
banana fritter		each		55
chow chow		1 portion		275
French				
beef bourguignon		1 portion		530
coq au vin		1 portion		650
duck in orange sauce		1 portion		720
escargots		1 portion		300
French onion soup		1 portion		280
mussels in wine sauce		1 portion		380
scallops in cheese sauce		1 portion		350
sole, grilled		1 portion		310
sole Veronique		1 portion		550
steak au poivre		1 portion		490
tournados rossini		1 portion		600
trout, grilled		1 portion		240

Food Category or Brand	Calories /100g	Portion Size /g	Calories /port

Desserts

Food	Portion	Calories/port
bombe	1 portion	180
chocolate gateau	1 portion	400
chocolate mousse	1 portion	260
crêpes Suzette	1 portion	400
pineapple in Kirsch	1 portion	90

Greek

Food	Portion	Calories/port
bean soup	1 portion	250
Greek salad	1 portion	180
houmous with pitta	1 portion	460
kalamari, deep fried	1 portion	500
kalamari, marinaded	1 portion	200
kebabs	1 portion	320
meatballs	1 portion	580
moussaka	1 portion	665
stifado	1 portion	565
stuffed vine leaves	1 portion	300
taramasalata with pitta	1 portion	450
tzatziki	1 portion	56

Desserts

Food	Portion	Calories/port
halva	1 portion	260
layered pastry (filo)	1 portion	360

Indian

Food	Portion	Calories/port
chapati	each	140
chicken curry	1 portion	745
chicken korma	1 portion	870
lamb biriyani	1 portion	920
meat Madras	1 portion	545
meat vindaloo	1 portion	565
mixed vegetable curry	1 portion	450
naan bread	each	300
onion bhaji, large	each	245

Food Category or Brand	Calories /100g	Portion	Size /g	Calories /port
pilau rice		1 portion		470
plain boiled rice		1 portion		310
poppadum		each		75
pork vindaloo		1 portion		595
potato curry		1 portion		515
prawn biriyani		1 portion		855
roghan ghosh		1 portion		720
samosa		each		260
tandoori chicken		1 portion		310
tomato sambal		1 portion		20
Desserts				
glub jamen		1 portion		365
kulfi		1 portion		215
mango slices		1 portion		155

Italian
Antipasti

Food Category or Brand	Calories /100g	Portion	Size /g	Calories /port
artichokes	379			
calf's liver with sage		1 portion		270
cannelloni		1 portion		500
lasagne		1 portion		650
mixed fish salad		1 portion		365
mixed fried fish		1 portion		1000
mixed vegetables	330			
mushrooms	381			
Parma ham with figs		1 portion		120
Parma ham with melon		1 portion		150
peppers	331			
ravioli		1 portion		510
scampi provençale		1 portion		500
spaghetti bolognese		1 portion		720
spaghetti carbonara		1 portion		1020
spaghetti marinara		1 portion		690
spaghetti napoletana		1 portion		630
spaghetti al pesto		1 portion		855

Food Category or Brand	Calories /100g	Portion	Size /g	Calories /port
squid		1 portion		300
stacciatelle		1 portion		100
stuffed tomatoes		1 portion		200
sun-dried tomatoes	387			

Desserts

cassata		1 portion		150
figs		1 portion		60
profiteroles		1 portion		600

Fast Foods

Most of the items in this listing come from the popular international food chains. These organizations practise 'portion control', so the calorie figures should be fairly accurate. If you are visiting a privately-owned fast food outlet, the figures given here should at least provide an indication of the calorie content of individual dishes on offer.

Here are some bits of advice for slimmers:

- hamburger places: if possible choose a hamburger by itself, without bun or French fries, accompanied by a simple salad. Avoid cheeseburgers and be aware that some barbecue sauces contain surprising amounts of sugar.
- chicken restaurants: ask for grilled or roast chicken instead of fried.
- fish and chips: again, ask for a salad rather than chips – and see if grilled fish is available rather than battered-and-fried.
- pizza restaurants: the problem isn't so much the pizza dough (though you'd do better to ask for the thin and crispy type of base) but the toppings. The basic pizza topping is cheese and tomato, of course – let cheese be

the only high-calorie element in the total mix. (See also the separate **Rice, Pasta and Pizza** section).
- **Sandwiches** are in their own section.
- Milk shakes can be found in **Drinks** (Non-alcoholic).

Food Category or Brand	Calories /100g	Portion	Size /g	Calories /port
Burger King				
Big King		each		537
Burger King flamer		each		308
cheeseburger		each		328
chicken Dinos (x4)		each		119
chicken Dinos (x6)		each		179
chicken royale		each		587
chicken royale club		each		618
deli wrap: cajun chicken		each		511
deli wrap: chicken caesar		each		484
double cheeseburger		each		489
double cheeseburger with bacon		each		506
double supreme		each		644
double whopper		each		821
double whopper with cheese		each		903
French fries, large				490
French fries, regular				400
French fries, small				259
hamburger		each		287
onion rings				261
spicy beanburger		each		505
veggie whopper		each		432
whopper		each		594
whopper junior		each		349
whopper junior with cheese		each		390
whopper with cheese		each		676

Food Category or Brand	Calories /100g	Portion	Size /g	Calories /port
Breakfasts				
bacon & egg		serving		296
egg & cheese		serving		282
hash browns large (18)		serving		318
hash browns medium (12)		serving		212
sausage & egg		serving		375
sausage, bacon & egg		serving		430
Desserts				
apple fritters		serving		157
birthday cake		each		389
choc chip cookie		each		79
chocolate topping		serving		38
cinnamon hot bakes		serving		399
diddy cones		each		92
diddy donut		serving		323
diddy donut – chocolate		serving		380
diddy donut – strawberry		each		378
double choc chip cookie		each		78
ice cream sundae caramel		serving		189
ice cream sundae chocolate		serving		189
soft serve ice cream		serving		112
strawberry topping		serving		38
toffee fudge topping		serving		46
vanilla ice-cream – tub		each		192
vanilla ice-cream – tub (with chocolate sauce)		each		194
vanilla ice-cream – tub (with strawberry sauce)		each		192
wafer cone		serving		48
Dips/Sauces				
bbq sauce pot		each		25
Dijon mayo sauce pot		each		112
garlic sauce dip pot		each		85

Food Category or Brand	Calories /100g	Portion	Size /g	Calories /port
hot chilli sauce pot		each		26
ketchup pot		each		25

Drinks

coca-cola, large		each		258
coca-cola, regular		each		172
coca-cola, small		each		129
coffee (black)		each		2
diet coke, large		each		6
diet coke, regular		each		4
diet coke, small		each		3
fanta orange, large		each		258
fanta orange, regular		each		172
fanta orange, small		each		129
hot chocolate		each		65
milk shake small banana		each		283
milk shake small chocolate		each		292
milk shake small strawberry		each		277
milk shake small vanilla		each		220
orange juice, freshly squeezed		each		123
orange juice minute maid		serving		120
sprite, large		each		258
sprite, regular		each		172
sprite, small		each		129
tea (white no sugar)		each		22

Carveries

Starters

avocado with prawns		1 serving		320
melon		1 serving		40
pâté on toast		1 serving		400
prawn cocktail		1 serving		270
tomato soup		1 serving		80
vegetable soup		1 serving		75

Food Category or Brand	Calories /100g	Portion	Size /g	Calories /port
Roast Meats				
beef, lean	220	1 serving	50	110
beef, lean & fat	320	1 serving	50	160
chicken	170	1 serving	50	85
chicken with skin	240	1 serving	50	120
lamb, lean	220	1 serving	50	110
lamb, lean & fat	300	1 serving	50	150
pork crackling		1 serving		65
pork, lean	160	1 serving	50	80
pork, lean & fat	320	1 serving	50	160
turkey	160	1 serving	50	80
turkey with skin	190	1 serving	50	95
Side Orders				
apple sauce		2 tbsp		40
bacon roll		each		25
gravy		2 tbsp		30
horseradish sauce		1 tsp		10
mint sauce		1 tbsp		5
Yorkshire pudding		1 serving		120
Desserts				
cheesecake		1 serving		390
crème caramel		1 serving		200
fresh fruit salad		1 serving		80
fruit pies, all flavours		1 serving		360
ice-cream, all flavours		2 scoops		225
sherry trifle		1 serving		410
sorbet with wafer		2 scoops		100
Fish & Chip Shops				
chicken in batter		1 portion		640
chips, average portion		1 portion		560
chips, large portion		1 portion		860
chips, small portion		1 portion		390

Food Category or Brand	Calories /100g	Portion	Size /g	Calories /port
cod in batter		1 portion		330
cod roe in batter		1 portion		200
gherkins, large		each		10
haddock in batter		1 portion		340
mushy peas		1 portion		140
plaice in batter		1 portion		650
rockfish in batter		1 portion		650
sausage in batter		1 portion		225
sausage, jumbo		each		250
saveloy		each		230
scampi in batter		1 portion		240
skate in batter		1 portion		460
tartare sauce		1 sachet		30
tomato ketchup		1 sachet		20
vinegar				0

Kentucky Fried Chicken

barbecue beans, regular		each		92
burger, cheese & bacon		each		515
chicken		1 piece		220
classic burger		each		420
classic burger & cheese		each		460
corn on the cob		each		180
corn salad, large		each		355
corn salad, regular		each		150
fillet burger		each		385
fillet burger & cheese		each		475
fillet burger, cheese & bacon		each		480
French fries, large		each		375
French fries, regular		each		295

Side Orders

American biscuit		each		335

Desserts

apple pie		each		250

Food Category or Brand	Calories /100g	Portion	Size /g	Calories /port
Little Chef				
Snacks				
BLT sandwich		each		630
chicken open sandwich		each		320
Starters				
chicken soup		1 serving		125
Mexican dipper		1 serving		405
mushroom dipper		1 serving		390
prawn cocktail		1 serving		260
salmon terrine		1 serving		215
tomato soup		1 serving		160
Salads				
coleslaw		1 serving		195
prawn salad		1 serving		555
side salad		1 serving		165
Main Dishes				
Big-7 beefburger		each		1070
Big-7 cheeseburger		each		1180
Big choice chicken		1 serving		805
cheese & ham tagliatelle		1 serving		710
chef's grill		1 serving		1355
chicken platter		1 serving		875
chipped potatoes		1 serving		410
fillet of cod		1 serving		705
fillet of haddock		1 serving		1015
gammon steak		1 serving		805
lemon sole fingers		1 serving		1055
liver & bacon grill		1 serving		1185
scampi platter		1 serving		985
steak platter		1 serving		1280
tagliatelle bolognese		1 serving		540
vegetarian tagliatelle		1 serving		495
whole plaice		1 serving		745

Food Category or Brand	Calories /100g	Portion	Size /g	Calories /port
Desserts				
cheesecake, all flavours		1 serving		345
chocolate Arctic ice		1 serving		440
chocolate fudge cake		1 serving		385
hot choc 'n' ice		1 serving		480
lemon sorbet		1 serving		100
mint Arctic ice		1 serving		385
pancakes with ice-cream		1 serving		365
raspberry Arctic ice		1 serving		305
sugar & lemon pancakes		1 serving		280
McDonalds				
Bacon McDouble with cheese		each		478
Big Mac		each		493
cheeseburger		each		299
chicken McNuggets (20)				843
chicken McNuggets (6)				253
chicken McNuggets (9)				380
filet-o-fish		each		389
French fries (large)				412
French fries (medium)				293
French fries (regular)				206
hamburger		each		253
McChicken sandwich		each		375
quarter pounder		each		423
quarter pounder with cheese		each		516
vegetable deluxe		each		423
Sauces				
barbeque		pot		55
mild mustard		pot		63
sweet & sour		pot		58
sweet curry		pot		61
tomato ketchup		pot		26
mayo		pot		180

Food Category or Brand	Calories /100g	Portion	Size /g	Calories /port
Desserts				
apple pie		each		230
birthday cake		each		250
donut – chocolate		each		329
donut – cinnamon		each		302
donut – sugared		each		303
ice-cream cone		each		157
ice-cream cone – with Cadbury's flake		each		204
McFlurry – with Crunchie		each		321
McFlurry – with Dairy Milk		each		280
McFlurry – with Smarties		each		327
sundae – hot caramel		each		358
sundae – hot fudge		each		351
sundae – strawberry		each		296
Drinks				
coca-cola (large)		each		226
coca-cola (medium)		each		172
coca-cola (regular)		each		108
coffee (with UHT creamer)		each		17
diet coke (large)		each		2
diet coke (medium)		each		2
diet coke (regular)		each		1
fanta orange (large)		each		226
fanta orange (medium)		each		172
fanta orange (regular)		each		108
hot chocolate drink		each		106
milk		each		124
milkshake – banana (large)		each		507
milkshake – banana (regular)		each		396
milkshake – chocolate (large)		each		516
milkshake – chocolate (regular)		each		403
milkshake – strawberry (large)		each		512
milkshake – strawberry (regular)		each		400
milkshake – vanilla (large)		each		490

Food Category or Brand	Calories /100g	Portion	Size /g	Calories /port
milkshake – vanilla (regular)		each		383
pure orange juice (large)		each		141
pure orange juice (regular)		each		94
sprite (large)		each		226
sprite (medium)		each		172
sprite (regular)		each		108
tea (with UHT skimmed milk)		each		10

Breakfast Menu

bacon & egg McMuffin		each		346
big breakfast		each		591
hash brown		each		138
muffin (buttered)		each		157
muffin (buttered) & preserve		each		234
pancakes & sausage		each		670
sausage & egg McMuffin		each		427

Perfect Pizza

Deep Pan, Medium

cheese & tomato		each		905
ham & mushroom		each		940
Hawaiian		each		970
meat feast		each		990
Mexican heatwave		each		1020
perfectionist		each		1085
vegetarian		each		920

Deep Pan, Large

cheese & tomato		each		1690
ham & mushroom		each		1765
Hawaiian		each		1825
meat feast		each		1860
Mexican heatwave		each		1925
perfectionist		each		2060
vegetarian		each		1725

Food Category or Brand	Calories /100g	Portion	Size /g	Calories /port
Thin Crust, Medium				
cheese & tomato		each		685
ham & mushroom		each		720
Hawaiian		each		755
meat feast		each		770
Mexican heatwave		each		800
perfectionist		each		870
vegetarian		each		705
Thin Crust, Large				
cheese & tomato		each		1275
ham & mushroom		each		1350
Hawaiian		each		1410
meat feast		each		1445
Mexican heatwave		each		1505
perfectionist		each		1645
vegetarian		each		1310
Pizza Express				
Antipizze				
baked dough balls		1 serving		200
bruschetta		1 serving		387
garlic bread		1 serving		278
mixed leaf salad		1 serving		190
mozzarella and tomato salad		1 serving		282
tonno e fagioli		1 serving		337
Salads				
Caesar salad		1 serving		298
mozzarella and tomato		1 serving		623
nicoise		1 serving		729
pollo		1 serving		573
Variations				
cannelloni		1 serving		531
ham & eggs		1 serving		504

Food Category or Brand	Calories /100g	Portion	Size /g	Calories /port
King Edward		1 serving		670
lasagne pasticciate		1 serving		500
melanzane Parmigiana		1 serving		645

Pizze

American		each		754
American hot		each		758
cajun		each		822
capricciosa		each		754
caprina		each		635
Fiorentina		each		724
four seasons		each		720
giardiniera		each		711
la reine		each		665
margherita		each		622
mushroom		each		627
Napoletana		each		650
Neptune		each		604
pizza alle noci		each		766
quattro formaggi		each		753
Siciliana		each		723
Sloppy Giuseppe		each		783
Soho Pizza		each		690
Veneziana		each		613

Desserts

anacleto bombe		1 serving		255
cassata		1 serving		192
cheesecake		1 serving		347
chocolate fudge cake		1 serving		395
duomo di bosco		1 serving		345
fresh fruit salad		1 serving		125
positano bombe		1 serving		176
ravello bombe		1 serving		246
tartufo		1 serving		292
tiramisu		1 serving		456
vanilla ice-cream		1 serving		119

Food Category or Brand	Calories /100g	Portion	Size /g	Calories /port
Pizza Hut				
Pan Pizza, Small				
sauce & cheese		each		715
seafood supreme		each		875
spicy hot one		each		780
super supreme		each		965
supreme		each		645
vegetarian		each		735
Thin 'n' Crispy, Small				
sauce & cheese		each		460
seafood supreme		each		685
spicy hot one		each		725
super supreme		each		760
supreme		each		645
vegetarian		each		620
Pastas				
lasagne		1 serving		530
spaghetti Bolognese		1 serving		395
tagliatelle supreme		1 serving		685
tagliatelle verdi vegetarian		1 serving		600
Salad				
mixed regular salad		1 serving		140
mixed regular salad with dressing		1 serving		330
Priazzos				
Florentine		each		1040
Roma		each		990
Verona		each		1000

Food Category or Brand	Calories /100g	Portion	Size /g	Calories /port
Pizzaland				
Deep Pan, 5-inch				
Caribbean		each		400
cheese & tomato		each		360
hot & spicy		each		400
passionara		each		510
seafood		each		415
spicy chicken		each		400
vegetable special		each		375
Deep Pan, 7-inch				
Caribbean		each		700
cheese & tomato		each		620
four seasons		each		775
hot & spicy		each		710
passionara		each		920
seafood		each		730
spicy chicken		each		700
vegetable special		each		650
Deep Pan, 10-inch				
Caribbean		each		1260
cheese & tomato		each		1100
four seasons		each		1400
hot & spicy		each		1275
passionara		each		1610
seafood		each		1325
spicy chicken		each		1260
vegetable special		each		1160
Traditional, 7-inch				
Caribbean		each		370
cheese & tomato		each		330
hot & spicy		each		370
passionara		each		485
seafood		each		385

Food Category or Brand	Calories /100g	Portion	Size /g	Calories /port
spicy chicken		each		370
vegetable special		each		345

Traditional, 10-inch
Caribbean		each		650
cheese & tomato		each		570
four seasons		each		720
hot & spicy		each		655
passionara		each		870
seafood		each		680
spicy chicken		each		650
vegetable special		each		600

Wimpy
chicken in a bun		each		530
fish & chips		1 serving		465
international grill		1 serving		730
Wimpy grill		1 serving		218

Desserts
chocolate nut sundae		each		230
fruit & nut sundae		each		235

Drinks
thick shake		each		250

Fats and Oils

Fats are solid; oils are liquid. In general, oils are high in polyunsaturates and fats have saturated and monounsaturated fats. Saturated fats can leave behind fatty deposits in the blood vessels; polyunsaturates, being more liquid, are less likely to do so – therefore polyunsaturates are considered more healthy for you.

All oils have about 900 kcal per 100 g, as do solid fats such as dripping and lard. All ordinary butters are about 740 kcal per 100 g; this is because they naturally obtain about 15 per cent water. Concentrated butter and ghee have had some of the water removed.

The various non-butter spreads usually consist of oil that has been hydrogenated and has had water added through various processes which the manufacturers try very hard to keep secret. Some non-butter spreads contain dairy by-products such as whey and dried butter milk. The many 'light' and 'reduced fat' varieties usually contain large amounts of water, sometimes in excess of 50 per cent; this is one reason why they are mostly unsuitable for cooking.

Margarines may be made either with animal and vegetable fats, or with vegetable fats alone. In general the soft margarines made from vegetable fats are the ones with the

highest proportion of polyunsaturates and the lowest levels
of cholesterol.

Food Category or Brand	Calories /100g
Generic Butter, Margarine & Other Solid Fats	
blended butter	740
concentrated butter	870
Cornish butter	740
country spread	685
Dutch unsalted butter	740
ghee	911
olive oil	900
pure beef dripping	900
pure lard	900
slightly salted butter	740
Branded Butter, Margarine & Other Solid Fats	
Dairy Crest	
Clover	689
Clover light	396
Willow	718
Delight	
extra low-fat spread	228
low-fat spread	386
Flora	
extra light sunflower	378
Iceland	
soft spread	596

Food Category or Brand	Calories /100g
Kraft	
Golden Churn	642
Mello, reduced fat	510
Mono	675
Utterly Butterly	630
Vitalite	639
Vitalite, light	349
Krona	
gold	646
silver	643
spreadable	553
Outline	
very low-fat spread	268
Safeway	
baking margarine	743
blended butter	737
Danish Butter	735
English butter	737
garlic butter	689
low-fat sunflower spread	386
olive reduced fat spread	536
savers blended spread	632
savers soft spread	545
soft margarine	729
soya margarine	736
sunflower light spread	358
sunflower savers	531
sunflower spread	634

Food Category or Brand	Calories /100g
Sainsbury's	
butter licious	628
creamy butter	734
economy reduced fat	536
economy sunflower	531
golden light	374
half fat butter spread	372
margarine for baking	738
olive gold, low fat	536
soft margarine	730
soya margarine	639
spreadable butter	738
sunflower margarine	634
sunflower margarine, light	499
St Ivel	
gold, light	365
gold, lowest	259
gold, unsalted	365
St Michael	
(Marks & Spencer)	
low fat butter spread	768
salted English butter	736
touch of butter	318
Stork	
light blend reduced fat	550

Food Category or Brand	Calories /100g
Tesco	
golden blend	678
half-fat sunflower spread	382
Waitrose	
English butter	737
light butter – half fat	370
soft tub margarine	634
soya spread	744
sunflower margarine	738
sunflower spread (low fat)	366
Generic Oils	
blended vegetable oil	900
corn oil	900
grapeseed oil	900
groundnut oil	900
hazelnut oil	900
olive oil	900
olive oil, extra virgin	900
olive oil, light	900
rapeseed oil	900
sesame oil	900
solid vegetable oil	900
soya oil	900
sunflower oil	900
walnut oil	900

Fish

Comparing the calorific value of various types or cuts of fish is not easy, as one 'serving' of some varieties will include the skin and bones, while for those types that can be filleted the whole portion is edible.

Looked at raw, a typical white fish – sole, plaice, halibut – would be 80 per cent water, 18 per cent protein and 1–2 per cent fat – and with no carbohydrate.

The typical raw 'fatty' or 'oily' fish – herring, for example – would be 64 per cent water, 17 per cent protein and 18 per cent fat (the balance is inedible). Depending on the season, some oily fish can contain up to 30 per cent fat.

Shell fish, like white fish, have relatively little fat.

White fish is best for slimming diets, but even the oily fish contain only polyunsaturated fats (unlike the fat found in animal meat) and are also rich in vitamins A and D.

If you're slimming, steaming or poaching fish adds few calories. Plain grilling is next best, then grilling with oil or butter, then deep-frying, and finally pan-frying. If fish are breaded, not only the breadcrumbs but the milk and egg used to bind them will add fats and carbohydrate to the dish.

Many branded products include fish in various sauces or in pies. These additional ingredients must be accounted for, particularly cheese or butter sauces, which will add calories in the form of fat.

Smoked or other forms of cured fish will contain less water, which means that, weight for weight, all nutrients will be more concentrated.

Fish can be canned in brine, tomato or oil – brine adds least to overall calorific value, tomato sauce most, oil somewhere in between.

The effects of marinating fish will depend on what's in the marinade – some contain sugars.

Food Category or Brand	Calories /100g	Portion	Size /g	Calories /port
Generic Fish				
abalone canned	146	1 serving	120	175
anchovies canned	143	1 serving	85	122
per fillet		1 fish		5
bass steamed	127	1 serving	85	108
steamed (with bone)	67	1 serving	120	80
bloaters grilled	255	1 serving	50	128
grilled (skin & bones)	189	1 serving	85	161
bream red, steamed	118	1 serving	85	100
steamed (with bones)	61	1 serving	120	73
sea, steamed (bones)	66	1 serving	120	79
brill steamed	115	1 serving	85	100
buckling fillets	214	1 serving	120	257
catfish fried	200	1 serving	85	170
fried (with bone)	188	1 serving	120	225
steamed (with bone)	100	1 serving	120	120
clams fresh, without shell	89	1 serving	120	107
cockles fresh	48	1 serving	85	40
cod fried	139	1 serving	85	120
fried in batter	203	1 serving	85	195
grilled	160	1 serving	85	135
grilled (skin & bones)	136	1 serving	100	135

Food Category or Brand	Calories /100g	Portion	Size /g	Calories /port
steamed	82	1 serving	85	70
steamed (skin & bones)	66	1 serving	120	80
cod roe baked in vinegar	128	1 serving	85	110
fried	206	1 serving	85	175
conger fried (with bones)	252	1 serving	100	255
steamed	110	1 serving	85	95
steamed (skin & bones)	83	1 serving	100	85
crab boiled	127	1 serving	85	105
boiled (with shell)	25	1 crab	105	
dabs fried (with bones)	199	1 serving	85	170
dogfish fried (with bones)	300	1 serving	85	255
eels silver, stewed	374	1 serving	85	320
fish cakes fried	171	2 cakes	85	145
fishfingers fried	175	5 fingers	85	150
fish paste	174	spread	10	20
flounder fried (with bones)	147	1 serving	120	175
steamed	95	1 serving	85	80
steamed (skin & bones)	53	1 serving	120	65
gurnet grey, steamed (skin & bones)	108	1 serving	120	130
red, steamed (skin & bones)	93	1 serving	120	110
haddock fresh, fried (skin & bone)	161	1 serving	120	190
fresh, steamed	97	1 serving	85	80
fresh, steamed (skin & bone)	74	1 serving	120	90
smoked, steamed	65	1 serving	120	80
hake steamed (skin & bones)	86	1 serving	120	105
halibut steamed	130	1 serving	85	110
steamed (skin & bones)	99	1 serving	120	120
herring baked (with bones)	174	1 serving	100	175
fried	235	1 serving	85	200
fried (with bones)	208	1 serving	100	210
herring roe fried	260	1 serving	85	220
John Dory steamed (skin & bones)	59	1 serving	100	60

Food Category or Brand	Calories /100g	Portion	Size /g	Calories /port
kippers baked	201	1 serving	85	170
baked (skin & bones)	108	1 serving	100	110
lemon sole fried (skin & bones)	173	1 serving	100	175
steamed	90	1 serving	85	75
steamed (skin & bones)	64	1 serving	100	65
ling fried (skin & bones)	186	1 serving	100	175
lobster boiled	119	1 serving	85	100
mackerel fried (skin & bones)	136	1 serving	100	135
monkfish fried (with bones)	145	1 serving	100	145
steamed (with bones)	79	1 serving	100	80
mullet grey, steamed (skin & bones)	81	1 serving	120	100
red, steamed (with bones)	85	1 serving	120	100
mussels boiled	87	1 serving	85	75
boiled (with shells)	26	1 serving	85	25
oysters raw	50	1 serving	85	43
pilchards canned	220	1 serving	85	185
plaice fried (with bones)	142	1 serving	100	140
steamed	92	1 serving	85	75
steamed (skin & bones)	50	1 serving	100	50
prawns cooked	104	1 serving	85	90
cooked (with shells)	40	1 serving	150	60
saithe steamed	98	1 serving	85	85
steamed (with bones)	83	1 serving	100	85
salmon canned (with liquid)	137	1 serving	85	115
fresh, steamed	199	1 serving	85	170
fresh, steamed (skin & bones)	161	1 serving	100	160
smoked	175	1 serving	85	150
sardines canned, oil	222	1 serving	50	150
canned, tomato	179	1 serving	50	90
scallops steamed	105	1 serving	85	90
shrimps cooked	114	1 serving	85	95
cooked (with shells)	38	1 serving	150	57

Food Category or Brand	Calories /100g	Portion	Size /g	Calories /port
smelts fried	408	1 serving	85	345
sole fried	274	1 serving	85	230
fried (with bones)	241	1 serving	120	290
steamed	84	1 serving	85	70
steamed (skin & bones)	50	1 serving	120	60
sprats bones & head, fresh, fried	390	1 serving	120	465
smoked, grilled	284	1 serving	120	340
sturgeon steamed (with bones)	105	1 serving	120	125
trout steamed (skin & bones)	88	1 serving	120	105
sea, steamed (skin & bones)	104	1 serving	120	125
tuna canned (in oil)	1300	1 serving	85	1105
canned, solids only	757	1 serving	85	645
turbot steamed	100	1 serving	85	85
steamed (skin & bones)	66	1 serving	120	80
whelks fresh	91	1 serving	85	80
with shells		each		14
whitebait fried	537	1 serving	50	270
whiting fried (skin & bones)	174	1 serving	120	210
steamed (skin & bones)	61	1 serving	120	75
winkles boiled	75	1 serving	120	90
boiled (with shell)		each		14

Branded Canned Fish
John West

cod roe, soft	84
dressed crab	143
dressed lobster	105
kipper fillets, oil	229
mackerel fillets, tomato	213
oysters, smoked	230
pilchards, brine	123
pilchards, tomato	135

Food Category or Brand	Calories /100g	Portion	Size /g	Calories /port
salmon, pink	155			
salmon, red	168			
sardines, tomato	220			
sild, tomato	180			
skippers, oil	243			
tuna, brine	113			
tuna, oil	189			
tuna, salad (3 bean mix)	222			
tuna, springwater	113			

Princes

anchovy fillets	198			
crab, brine	75			
crab, dressed	126			
herring, marinaded	178			
pilchards, tomato	135			
tuna chunks, brine	105			
tuna chunks, oil	195			
tuna flakes, brine	95			
tuna flakes, oil	221			
tuna steaks, brine	105			

Branded Frozen/Chilled Fish
Asda

breaded scampi	204			
cod fillets	89			
crab flavour sticks	113			
fish fingers	200			
haddock fillet in crispy batter	242			
smoked haddock fillets	101			
tiger prawns	107			
whitefish portions	192			

Food Category or Brand	Calories /100g	Portion	Size /g	Calories /port
Birds Eye				
Captain's cod pie	127			
cod fish finger		each		53
cod mornay	153			
cod steak in butter sauce	104			
cod steak in cheese sauce	96			
cod steak in crunch crumbs		each		225
cod steak in parsley sauce	89			
haddock fish finger		each		50
kipper fillets, buttered	205			
oven crispy cod	212			
salmon fish cake		each		85
smoked haddock	85			
value fish cake		each		90
Iceland				
cod bake		1 serving		297
cod bites		each		34
cod crumble		1 serving		485
Safeway				
chunky cod fillets	80			
cod fillets	80			
crab fish sticks	90			
king tiger prawns	100			
mackerel fillets	220			
monkfish tail fillets	81			
peeled prawns	73			
sardines	165			
whole prawns	94			
Sainsbury's				
chunky cod fillets		each		289
cod burgers		each		249
cod fish fingers		each		55

Food Category or Brand	Calories /100g	Portion	Size /g	Calories /port
cod in butter sauce		each		184
cod in parsley sauce		each		158
cod nuggets		1/2 pack		215
haddock fishcake		each		142
haddock portion (crumb)		each		255
salmon en croute		each		534
salmon fillet (crumb)		each		283
salmon fish cakes		each		187
smoked salmon pâté		1/2 pot		107
tuna pâté		1/2 pot		179

St Michael (Marks & Spencer)

cod	80
cod crumb	206
chunky haddock batter	169
chunky plaice crumb	172
fish fingers	186
haddock	74
haddock batter	210
haddock crumb	201
hake crumb	215
king prawn	68
kipper	206
lemon sole crumb	225
lemon sole goujons	221
plaice	80
plaice crumb	207
salmon fillets	200
scampi in crumb	180

Waitrose

anchovy fillets	472
crab sticks	94
haddock cutlets	75
halibut	103

Food Category or Brand	Calories /100g	Portion	Size /g	Calories /port
mackerel fillets in brine	222			
mackerel fillets in tomato	244			
pink salmon	171			
plaice	79			
rainbow trout	125			
red salmon	171			
sardines in soya oil	370			
sardines in tomato	209			
sardines with hot pepper	301			
scampi in crispy crumbs	195			
tuna in brine	113			
tuna in oil	207			

Young's

cod & parsley croquettes	192			
cod & prawn pies	195			
fish kebabs, fresh	56			
fish kebabs, smoked	134			
fisherman's pie	134			
fresh cod fishcakes	213			
garlic prawns	75			
lemon sole fillets	82			
microwave ocean pie	130			
ocean pie	110			
oriental prawns	110			
sea scallops	93			
smoked haddock fillets	87			
trout amande	160			

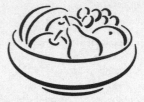

Fruit

Fresh fruit is between 80 and 90 per cent water. Most of the energy fruit provides is in the form of sugar – glucose, fructose (a form of sugar peculiar to fruit) and sucrose. Bananas and grapes have, among the fruits commonly available, the highest proportion of sugars.

The actual amount of sugar in any fruit depends on when it was picked. Most fruits do not contain significant amounts of fat, though there are some notable exceptions – olives, with up to 20 per cent for some varieties, and avocados, which are usually also around 15 to 20 per cent but can be as much as 40 per cent.

Fruit oils are, of course, polyunsaturated.

Although this book is only about the calorific values of foods, it's worth mentioning that fruit is, of course, an extremely good source of vitamin C.

Stewing is the most common method of cooking fruit. As a rough guide, the effect of adding a normal amount of sugar to the water used for stewing is to multiply by $2^{1}/_{2}$–3 the calorific value of a portion: apples stewed without sugar end up at 25 kcal/100 g; with added sugar in stewing they are 74 kcal/100 g.

In a dried fruit, such as apricots, the water constituent drops from around 85 per cent down to 25 per cent; all the other values obviously increase in proportion. By the time they are reconstituted, the water proportion is back to about 65 per cent. Many people would add sugar when they reconstitute: if no sugar is added, a 100 g portion would contain about 85 calories; once sugar is added, the portion contains 120 to 125 calories.

Most canned fruit is sunk into syrup rather than juice. This added syrup usually at least doubles the calorific value per portion.

Crystallized fruit is made by dipping fruit into a hot sugar solution. If you are slimming, avoid at all costs!

Food Category or Brand	Calories /100g	Portion	Size /g	Calories /port
Generic Fruits				
Apples				
cooking, baked (flesh only)	39	1 serving	130	50
cooking, baked (with skin)	31	1 serving	150	45
cooking, raw	37	1 apple	200	75
cooking, stewed (no sugar)	28	1 serving	150	45
eating (flesh only)	47	1 serving	130	60
eating (skin & core)	35	1 apple	185	65
Apricots				
canned, in syrup	106	1 serving	85	90
dried, no soak	125			
dried, stewed (no sugar)	61	1 serving	85	50
fresh	28	3 fruit	95	30
fresh (with stone)	26	3 fruit	120	30
fresh, stewed (no sugar)	22	1 serving	100	20

Food Category or Brand	Calories /100g	Portion	Size /g	Calories /port
Babaco				
flesh only	43	1 serving	130	
whole fruit, no seeds		1 fruit		195
Bananas				
fresh	77	1 banana		100
with skin	45	1 banana		100
Bilberries				
raw & frozen	57	1 serving	100	
Blackberries				
raw	30	1 serving	100	30
stewed (no sugar)	23	1 serving	100	23
Blackcurrants				
canned, in syrup	82	1 serving	100	82
raw & frozen	28	1 serving	100	28
stewed, no sugar	25	1 serving	100	25
Blueberries				
raw & frozen	64	1 serving	100	64
Cherries				
cooking, raw (with stones)	39	1 serving	100	39
raw (with stones)	40	1 serving	100	40
stewed (without sugar)	35	1 serving	100	35
Cranberries				
jelly	143	1 tbsp		25
raw	14	1 serving	100	
sauce	15	1/2 cup		200
Currants				
black, raw	29			

Food Category or Brand	Calories /100g	Portion	Size /g	Calories /port
black, stewed (no sugar)	22			
dried	244			
red, raw	21			
red, stewed (no sugar)	16			
white, raw	26			
white, stewed (no sugar)	20			
Damsons				
raw (with stones)	34	1 serving	100	34
stewed, no sugar (stones)	29	1 serving	100	29
Dates				
dried	272			
fresh	248	1 serving	100	248
fresh, with stones	214	1 serving	120	255
Figs				
dried, raw	214	1 serving	50	110
dried, stewed (no sugar)	107	1 serving	100	110
green	41	1 serving	100	40
Fruit Salad				
canned, in syrup	94	1 serving	120	110
Ginger Stem				
canned, in syrup	214	1 serving	120	257
Gooseberries				
green, raw	17			
ripe	37	1 serving	120	45
stewed (no sugar)	13	1 serving	120	15
Grapefruit				
fresh	22	½ grapefruit		45
with skin & pips	11	½ grapefruit		23

Food Category or Brand	Calories /100g	Portion	Size /g	Calories /port
Grapes				
black (skin, pips & stalks)	51	1 serving	150	75
white (skin, pips & stalks)	60	1 serving	150	90
Greengages				
fresh, with stones	45	1 serving	120	55
stewed, no sugar (stones)	37	1 serving	120	45
Guava				
canned	61	1 serving	85	52
fresh	57	1 serving	120	68
Kiwi				
fresh	107			
Kumquat				
fresh	64	1 serving	120	
whole fruit		1 fruit		5
Lemons				
juice	7	glass	100	5
whole fruit	15	1 fruit	100	15
Loganberries				
canned, in syrup	101	1 serving	110	100
fresh	17	1 serving	120	20
stewed (no sugar)	13	1 serving	120	15
Lychee				
canned	68	1 serving	110	74
fresh	28	1 fruit	50	14
Mandarins				
canned	64	glass	100	65
fresh (with skin)	45	1 mandarin		50

Food Category or Brand	Calories /100g	Portion	Size /g	Calories /port
Mango				
raw, flesh only	61	1 serving	120	73
Mangosteen				
whole fruit	71	1 fruit	65	20
Medlars				
flesh	43	1 serving	120	52
Melons				
cantaloupe (flesh)	24	½ melon	130	55
cantaloupe (with skin)	15	½ melon	360	55
charentais (flesh)	11	½ melon	300	33
honeydew	13	½ melon	300	39
ogen	15	½ melon	300	45
water (flesh)	54	wedge	300	162
yellow (with skin)	13	½ melon	300	40
Mulberries				
fresh	36			
Nectarines				
fresh (with stones)	46	1 serving	120	55
Olives				
with stones	85	1 serving	85	70
Oranges				
fresh	35	1 orange	140	50
fresh, with peel & pips	27	1 orange	185	50
juice, canned	217			
juice, from concentrate	157			
juice, fresh	38	glass	150	55
juice, frozen, diluted	45	glass	150	65

Food Category or Brand	Calories /100g	Portion /g	Size /port	Calories
Ortaniques				
flesh	57			
flesh with skin	43			
whole fruit		1 fruit	142	60
Passion Fruit				
with skin	15			
Papaw (Papaya)				
fresh, flesh only	39	1 serving	110	43
Peaches				
canned, in syrup	87	1 serving	100	87
dried, raw	213			
dried, stewed (no sugar)	70	1 serving	100	70
fresh	37	1 peach	110	40
fresh (with stones)	32	1 peach	125	40
Pears				
canned, in syrup	77	1 serving	120	90
cooking, raw (fresh)	36			
cooking, stewed (no sugar)	27	1 serving	120	35
eating, fresh	40	1 pear	175	70
eating, flesh (incl. core)	30	1 pear	350	70
Pineapple				
canned, in syrup	77	1 serving	100	77
fresh	46	1 serving	100	46
Plums				
cooking, raw, fresh (skins)	26			
cooking, raw (with stones)	23	1 serving	120	25
dessert, raw	38	1 plum		20
desserts, raw (stones)	36	1 plum		20
stewed, no sugar (stones)	20	1 serving	120	25

Food Category or Brand	Calories /100g	Portion /g	Size /port	Calories
Pomegranate				
juice	44	glass	100	44
Prunes				
dried, raw, pitted	161			
dried, raw (with stones)	134			
stewed, no sugar (stones)	81	1 serving	100	81
Quinces				
fresh	25			
Raisins				
dried	247			
Raspberries				
raw	25	1 serving	120	30
stewed (no sugar)	23	1 serving	100	23
Rhubarb				
stewed (no sugar)	5	1 serving	120	10
Sharon Fruit				
fresh	78	1 serving	100	
whole fruit		1 fruit		130
Strawberries				
fresh (no stalk)	26	1 serving	120	30
Sultanas				
dried	249			
Tangerines				
fresh	34	1 tangerine	120	40
with peel & pips	24	1 tangerine	120	30

Food Category or Brand	Calories /100g	Portion /g	Size /port	Calories
Topaz				
flesh only	57	1 serving	120	
flesh & skin	39	1 serving	120	
whole fruit		1 fruit		65
Ugli Fruit				
flesh only	53	1 serving	120	
flesh & skin	36	1 serving	120	
whole fruit		1 fruit		140

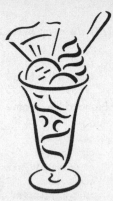

Ice-cream

Commercial ice-creams are made from milk, cream, milk products, non-milk fats, flavourings, stabilizers and emulsifiers. The other big ingredient is sugar.

'Dairy' ice-creams must contain at least 5 per cent milk fat and must not contain any other sort of fat (except that found in egg yolk). The luxury dairy ice-creams often contain 15 or more per cent milk fat/cream. In 'non-dairy' ice-creams, other fats, such as vegetable oils may be used.

All ice-cream contains air as part of its structure – soft ice-cream contains more air than traditional types. In a traditional dairy ice-cream, half of its volume is air.

Water accounts for about 60 to 70 per cent of an ice-cream's weight, protein about 4 per cent, fat about 10 per cent (mostly saturated and monounsaturated) and carbohydrate (nearly all sugar) just under 25 per cent. Some flavoured ice-creams have considerably more sugar.

A sorbet or water ice will usually have, weight for weight, half the calories of a dairy ice. There's no milk, cream or other oil, of course – but there *is* plenty of sugar.

Mousses appear in the **Desserts** section.

A serving is 100 g, unless stated otherwise.

Food Category or Brand	Calories /100g	Portion	Size /g	Calories /port
Branded Ice-creams				
Asda				
blackcurrant	101			
choc ices	265			
chocolate soft scoop	173			
cornish dairy	195			
really fruity tropical sorbet	125			
rocket lollies	56			
strawberry ice-cream cone	263			
toffee fudge soft scoop	185			
vanilla soft scoop	142			
Ben & Jerry's				
butter almond toffee	282			
choc chip cookie dough	260			
choc fudge brownie	260			
chunky monkey	283			
cool Britannia	250			
rainforest chunk	293			
Bertorelli				
cassata bombe dairy	215	1 bombe		614
chocolate dairy	211			
chocolate menthe	233			
coffee	196			
lemon surprise	225			
lemon water ice	109			
mela menthe	306	each		213
mela parisienne	302	each		211
mela stragata	298	each		208
orange surprise	220			
orange water ice	110			
praline dairy	210			
raspberry water ice	101			
strawberry dairy	176			
vanilla dairy	202			

Food Category or Brand	Calories /100g	Portion	Size /g	Calories /port
Birds Eye Wall's				
Bart Simpson – caramel swirl		each		172
calippo mini		each		60
calippo orange/tropical/ strawberry		each		100
chunky choc ice		each		163
cornetto choc 'n' nut		each		220
cornetto mint choc chip		each		215
cornetto strawberry		each		190
cornetto whippy		each		230
cream of cornish		each tub	125	95
feast chocolate		each		315
feast mini (chocolate)		each		195
feast mini (toffee)		each		190
feast toffee		each		310
magnum almond		each		330
magnum caramel and nuts		each		206
magnum classic		each		295
magnum double caramel		each		390
magnum double chocolate		each		371
magnum mint		each		295
magnum white		each		300
mini milk (chocolate/ strawberry/vanilla)		each		35
orange fruity		each		75
solero (exotic or summer)		each		130
solero ice		each		80
solero ice minis		each		65
twister		each		90
SOFT SCOOP				
vanilla	230			
vanilla light	180			

Food Category or Brand	Calories /100g	Portion	Size /g	Calories /port
CARTE D'OR				
coconut	240			
crème caramel	256			
strawberry	250			
triple chocolate	250			
vanilla	320			
VIENNETTA				
banana chocolate	150			
chocolate	260			
lemon	260			
mint	260			
original	300			
strawberry cheesecake	310			
TOO GOOD TO BE TRUE				
chocolate	180			
vanilla	150			
Häagen-Dazs				
choc choc chip	265			
macadamia nut brittle	263			
praline & cream	276			
strawberry	280			
vanilla	260			
Iceland				
black cherry & Kirsch	169			
cassata	165			
chocolate 'n' nut	225			
chocolate orange (Cointreau)	169			
crunchy toffee	201			
ice-cream roll		1/6 roll		82
mint chocolate chip	169			
neapolitan	165			

Food Category or Brand	Calories /100g	Portion	Size /g	Calories /port
neapolitan chequers	162			
passion fruit & peach	179			
raspberry ripple	169			
strawberry vanilla bombe		whole		193
vanilla (economy)	123			
white vanilla	158			
CHOC ICES				
chocolate 'n' nut		1 choc ice		119
dark mint		1 choc ice		115
chocolate 'n' nut cornet		1 cornet		258
chocolate 'n' nut sundae		1 sundae		177

Loseley

acacia honey & ginger	188			
apricot sorbet	79			
blackcurrant sorbet	69			
Brazilian mocha	212			
lemon sorbet	67			
Montezuma chocolate	167			
passion fruit	66			
pineapple sorbet	74			
sovereign strawberry	160			
vanilla, old-fashioned	202			
woodland hazel	200			

Lyons Maid

COCKTAIL

Blue Hawaiian		each		34
Brandy Alexander		each		81
Piña Colada		each		60

CUTTING BRICKS

chocolate ripple	181			
neapolitan	179			

Food Category or Brand	Calories /100g	Portion	Size /g	Calories /port
peach Melba	177			
raspberry ripple	173			
vanilla	182			
GOLD SEAL				
caramel toffee	210			
chocolate coconut flake	183			
chocolate swirl	192			
mint chocolate chip	196			
rum & raisin	184			
vanilla chocolate flake	219			

St Michael (Marks & Spencer)

chocolate sundae	247			
Cornish blackberry	218			
Cornish strawberry	229			
giant chocolate cone	279			
giant strawberry cone	263			
milk chocolate ices	306			
organic chocolate	255			
organic vanilla	220			
vanilla soft scoop	180			

Ross

chocolate	180			
chocolate ripple	180			
Cornish dairy	160			
raspberry ripple	170			
strawberry	170			
vanilla	170			
vanilla choc ices	157	1 choc ice		102

Safeway

gold rush banoffee	242			
lemon pavlova	191			

Food Category or Brand	Calories /100g	Portion	Size /g	Calories /port
misty mountain blue	240			
neapolitan	172			
raspberry ripple	161			
strawberry scandal	174			
toffee temptation	221			
Sainsbury's				
chocolate	164			
lemon sorbet	120			
neapolitan	160			
raspberry pavlova	207			
raspberry ripple	161			
vanilla	162			
Waitrose				
assorted lollies	51			
assorted splits	108			
butter toffee soft	227			
cookies & cream	161			
dairy strawberry	217			
dark choc ices	303			
luxury clotted cream	271			
mango sorbet	89			
maple & almond	265			
raspberry ripple	197			
rum & raisin	134			
soft vanilla ice	93			
tropical fruit sorbet	95			
white chocolate	208			
Weight Watchers				
neapolitan	93	serving		68
vanilla	96	serving		69

Jams, Spreads, Sauces and Pickles

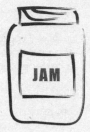

A true jam, made properly with sugar as a preservative, is usually about 250 kcal per 100 g; 70 g of that will be carbohydrate in the form of sugar. In a reduced-sugar formula, the carbohydrate content may be only 30 to 35 g out of the total 100 and the calorific value will be down to around 125.

The really high-calorie spreads are the nut spreads (except for peanut butter), particularly those that also contain chocolate. A hazelnut chocolate spread can contain, weight for weight, more than twice the calories of a regular fruit jam.

Butter is listed in the **Fats and Oils** section; pâtés can be found in the sections on **Fish** and **Meat and Poultry**; cheese spreads are in the **Dairy Products** section.

The calorific value of pickles usually depends on the amount of sugar used in the pickling brine.

Food Category or Brand	Calories /100g	Portion	Size /g	Calories /port

Branded Jams and Spreads
Baxters

jams, reduced sugar, all types	210			
marmalade, all types	210			

Cadbury's

chocolate spread	315			
hazelnut chocolate spread	570			

Chivers

lemon curd	285			
marmalade, all types	255			

Cross & Blackwell

redcurrant jelly	259			

Ferrero

Nutella	525			

Gales

honey, all types	310			
lemon curd	280			
peanut butter	586			

Hartley's

jelly jams	260			
lemon cheese	295			
marmalade	255			
mincemeat	285			
pure fruit jams	255			

Heinz

celery, corn & apple	188			
cucumber sandwich	185			
speciality tangy sandwich	133			
speciality mild mustard	128			

Food Category or Brand	Calories /100g	Portion	Size /g	Calories /port
Marmite				
		1 teasp.		13
Princes Pastes				
beef	186			
chicken & ham	226			
crab	107			
salmon	196			
sardine & tomato	118			
tuna	209			
Robertson's				
jams, all flavours	251			
lemon curd	291			
marmalade, all types	251			
mincemeat, all flavours	266			
pure fruit spreads, all flavours	120			
Safeway				
REDUCED SUGAR				
apricot	186			
blackcurrant	174			
marmalade	185			
raspberry	182			
strawberry	188			
St Michael (Marks & Spencer)				
apricot conserve	237			
blackcurrant conserve	237			
Canadian honey	300			
lemon & lime marmalade	254			
lemon curd	304			
maple syrup	266			
raspberry conserve	246			
shredless marmalade	260			

Food Category or Brand	Calories /100g	Portion	Size /g	Calories /port
strawberry conserve	236			
toffee sauce	336			

Spar
conserves, all types	247			

Sun-Pat
hazelnut chocolate spread	526			
peanut butter	174			
wholenut peanut butter	175			

Waitrose
apricot conserve	262			
apricot spread (no added sugar)	133			
blackcurrant	262			
blackcurrant jelly	264			
grapefruit marmalade	266			
Greek honey	305			
honey, clear	305			
lemon curd	301			
orange marmalade	264			
pure honey, set	305			
raspberry	258			
raspberry conserve	258			
strawberry spread (no added sugar)	138			
thick cut marmalade	265			

Generic Sauces & Pickles
mayonnaise (low-calorie)	350			
mayonnaise (regular)	725			

Food Category or Brand	Calories /100g	Portion	Size /g	Calories /port

Branded Sauces & Pickles

Baxters

apple	49			
cranberry jelly	268			
creamy four cheese	104			
creamy mushroom	92			
horseradish sauce	326			
mango with ginger chutney	187			
mint jelly	264			
redcurrant jelly	260			
seafood sauce	533			
tartare sauce	515			

Coleman's

MUSTARDS

English	187			
American	110			
Dijon	170			
French mild	104			
German	135			
horseradish	140			
mild burger	110			
wholegrain	173			
honey	208			

CONDIMENTS

bramley apple sauce	108			
hot horseradish	105			
lemon & tarragon	287			
mint sauce	112			
seafood sauce	335			
tartare	263			

Food Category or Brand	Calories /100g	Portion	Size /g	Calories /port
Safeway				
95% fat free Italian	86			
95% fat free onion, garlic & herb	83			
balti	375			
blue cheese	462			
cajun	346			
guacamole	229			
houmous	309			
houmous, reduced fat	249			
onion & chives	429			
pesto	359			
salsa	57			
salsa (fresh)	64			
satay	324			
smoked bbq	329			
sour cream & chives	522			
sweet & sour	314			
taramasalata	449			
thousand island	512			
tikka	392			
Sainsbury's				
barbeque sauce		serving	15	18
bramley apple sauce	102			
brown sauce	117			
cocktail cherries	170			
Dijon mustard		teaspoon		8
French mayonnaise		serving	15	103
French vinaigrette		serving	10	40
fruit sauce		serving	15	16
horseradish sauce	98			
hot & cold Hollandaise sauce		serving	15	78
hot & cold mustard sauce		serving	15	64
Italian vinaigrette		serving	10	38
low fat thousand island dressing		serving	10	9

Food Category or Brand	Calories /100g	Portion	Size /g	Calories /port
mango chutney		serving	15	35
midget gherkins		serving	30	10
onion relish		serving	15	22
peach chutney		serving	15	28
piccalilli	228			
pickled onions		serving	50	17
pickled red cabbage		serving	50	20
reduced calorie French mayonnaise		serving	15	55
sauerkraut		serving	50	15
silverskin onions		serving	30	6
sweet pickle		serving	15	21
sweetcorn relish		serving	15	22
tomato & chilli relish		serving	15	20
tomato ketchup		serving	15	18
tomato relish		serving	15	20
whole baby beets		serving	50	29

St Michael (Marks & Spencer)

Food Category or Brand	Calories /100g
American bbq sauce	145
apple	49
caesar dressing	455
cocktail gherkins	32
cranberry sauce	190
Dijon mustard	153
English mustard	226
French dressing	570
French dressing lite	60
honey & mustard marinade	240
horseradish	313
Italian dressing	660
mango chutney	219
mayonnaise	740
mayonnaise lite	265
olives green	102
piccalilli	105

Food Category or Brand	Calories /100g	Portion	Size /g	Calories /port
pickled cucumbers	40			
pickled onions	42			
salad cream	391			
salsa	100			
seafood dressing	571			
tomato ketchup	120			

Waitrose

chilli sauce	27			
cocktail gherkins	9			
Cumberland sauce	274			
curried fruit chutney	176			
dark soy sauce	71			
garlic mayonnaise	702			
green olives in brine	196			
horseradish hot sauce	129			
lemon mayonnaise	698			
mango chutney	175			
mayonnaise	702			
mint sauce	120			
mustard piccalilli	56			
olives with garlic & chilli	487			
pickled beetroot	32			
pickled onions	32			
salad cream	318			
salsa	74			
sweet pickle	140			
tartare sauce	285			

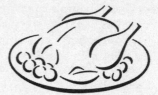

Meat and Poultry

Meat

Some cuts of meat include bone, skin, gristle and other inedible elements, so computing their exact calorific content can be a bit difficult.

Beef (without bone) will be about two-thirds water, 18 to 24 per cent protein and 10 to 20 per cent fat. The visible fat is mostly saturated, but all meats have veins of fat running through the flesh as well. The amount of visible fat may vary from 50 to 60 per cent (in the case of streaky bacon) down to below 20 per cent for so-called 'lean' meats. A great deal of the flavour of meat comes from the fat.

In general terms there is very little nutritional difference between various cuts from the same animal – the more expensive ones will be the most tender, while the cheaper ones will require slow cooking over a low heat or marinating to soften the tissues up. Of course, certain portions come with more fat attached, but this is partly a function of how the butcher has divided the cuts.

Pork is the fattiest meat commonly eaten, followed by lamb and then beef.

As far as cooking methods are concerned, the following would be the order of preference for someone who wants to minimize his or her fat intake: grilling (without basting), roasting (again without too much basting or using additional fats), boiling, simmering, stewing (where the cooking liquid is retained as part of the dish), frying. There are of course exceptions: oxtail is stewed and the liquid retained, but most cooks would skim the fat from the liquid before serving.

The weight of some frozen meat joints, particularly bacon and its relatives, is sometimes artificially boosted with additional water. The weights given here for frozen meat do not include this additional water.

Sausages, salamis and the like can be found in the **Processed Meats** section.

Poultry

The calorific value of poultry also depends largely on how much fat is on the meat. We can compare poultry that has been roasted: roast turkey is between 2 and 3 per cent fat, roast chicken between 5 and 6 per cent fat, roast grouse 5 per cent, partridge 7 per cent, pheasant 9 per cent, duck 10 per cent fat, pigeon 13 per cent and goose 22 per cent. Most of the fats found in poultry are monounsaturated and saturated. The remainder of the energy in poultry comes from meat proteins.

Fats add to the flavour of poultry and, especially in the case of turkey, the lack of fat can sometimes result in meat that is unacceptably dry – which is why most people lay strips of bacon over their turkey when they roast it.

The weight of some frozen poultry is artificially boosted by the injection of additional water.

The low-fat cooking methods are boiling (with the fluid discarded), grilling and barbecuing, tandoor cooking, roasting (with minimal basting and no additional fats) and stewing. Frying will inevitably add both carbohydrates and fat – the breadcrumbs provide the carbohydrates, the binder provides fat, and of course the cooking fat gets absorbed as well.

Increasingly, chicken and turkey are being offered in manufactured forms, such as pre-prepared roasts, or cuts cooked in Italian, Chinese or Indian style. You can also get shaped and breaded escalopes, frozen 'boneless joints' (in which turkey meat is surrounded with a layer of pork fat), and a number of derivatives of chicken kiev in which a pocket of meat is filled with butter and garlic (the classic kiev recipe) or various sauce/cheese/vegetable combinations. Inevitably the butter and cheese increase the fat – and cholesterol. See the **Ready-made Meals** section.

Look in the **Fast Foods** section for information about fried chicken take-away.

Food Category or Brand	Calories /100g	Portion	Size /g	Calories /port
Generic Meat				
Beef				
corned beef	231	1 slice	30	75
silverside, boiled	301	1 serving	85	190
sirloin, roast, lean	224	1 serving	85	190
sirloin, roast, lean & fat	385	1 serving	85	325
steak, fried	273	1 serving	85	230
steak, grilled	304	1 serving	85	260
steak, stewed	206	1 serving	85	175
topside, boiled	213	1 serving	85	180
topside, roast, lean	249	1 serving	85	210
topside, roast, lean & fat	321	1 serving	85	270
Veal				
calf's brain, boiled	103	1 serving	100	103
calf's liver, fried	262	1 serving	85	220

Food Category or Brand	Calories /100g	Portion	Size /g	Calories /port
cutlet, fried	215	1 serving	85	185
fillet, roast	231	1 serving	85	195
Brawn	153	1 serving	120	
Hare				
roast	193	1 serving	85	165
roast, with bone	131	1 serving	100	131
stewed	194	1 serving	85	165
stewed, with bone	142	1 serving	100	142
Also see Rabbit				
Luncheon Meats				
canned	335	1 serving	85	295
meat paste	173	spread	20	35
Mutton				
chop, grilled, lean	271	1 serving	90	240
chop, grilled, lean without bone	127	1 serving	120	150
chop, grilled, lean & fat without bone	378	1 serving	120	450
chop, fried, lean & fat without bone	512	1 serving	120	615
leg, boiled	260	1 serving	100	260
leg, roast	292	1 serving	100	326
scrag & neck, stewed	326	1 serving	100	326
scrag & neck, stewed without bone	245	1 serving	120	295
sheep's brain, boiled	110	1 serving	100	110
sheep's heart, roast	239	1 serving	85	205
sheep's kidney, fried	199	1 serving	85	170
sheep's tongue, stewed	296	1 serving	85	250

Food Category or Brand	Calories /100g	Portion	Size /g	Calories /port
Ox				
kidney, stewed	159	1 serving	25	40
liver, fried	284	1 serving	85	240
tail, stewed	250	1 serving	85	
tail, stewed with bones	89	1 serving	85	
tongue, pickled	309	1 serving	85	260
Pork				
chops, grilled, lean	325	1 serving	85	275
chops, grilled, lean with bone	133	1 serving	100	133
chops, grilled, lean & fat with bone	451	1 serving	100	451
leg roast	317	1 serving	100	317
loin, roast, lean	284	1 serving	100	284
loin, roast, lean & fat	455	1 serving	100	455
loin, salt, smoked lean	243	1 serving	100	243
Bacon				
fried, back	597	2 slices	25	150
fried, collar	438	2 slices	25	110
fried, streaky	526	2 slices	25	130
Gammon				
boiled, lean	193	1 serving	100	
boiled, lean & fat	325	1 serving	100	
rashers, fried	432	2 slices	20	
rashers, grilled	403	2 slices	20	
Ham				
boiled, lean	219	1 serving	85	185
boiled, lean & fat	435	1 serving	85	370
chopped	340	1 serving	85	290

Food Category or Brand	Calories /100g	Portion	Size /g	Calories /port
Rabbit				
stewed	180	1 serving	85	150
stewed with bone	92	1 serving	120	110
Also see Hare				
Sweetbreads				
stewed	177	1 serving	85	150
Tripe				
stewed	102	1 serving	100	102
Venison				
roast	196	1 serving	85	165
Branded Meat Products				
Bowyers				
brawn	243			
chopped ham	275			
haslet	289			
pork shoulder	161			
prime ham	161			
stuffed pork roll	325			
Butterball				
beef grillsteak		each		245
Dipper		each		60
Cherry Valley				
confit de canard	225		400	900
Iceland				
bacon burger		each		100
beef sandwich steak		each		320
chilli beef crispbake		each		195
Chinese ribsteaks	178			

Food Category or Brand	Calories /100g	Portion	Size /g	Calories /port
corned beef crispbake		each		195
lamb grillsteak		each		205
ribsteaks	178			
Stilton & bacon chicken		each		330

Mr Brain's

faggots in rich sauce		each		130

Sainsbury's

chopped pork and ham	267	can		908
cooked lean ham	100	can		113
English premium ham		slice		34
honey roast ham		slice		33
lean cooked ham		slice		121
peppered ham		slice		32
smoked ham		slice		18

Generic Poultry
Chicken

boiled	203	1 serving	85	170
boiled, with bone	132	1 serving	100	132
roast	189	1 serving	85	160
roast, with bone	102	1 serving	100	102

Duck

roast	313	1 serving	85	265
roast, with bone	169	1 serving	100	169

Goose

roast	323	1 serving	85	275
roast, with bone	187	1 serving	100	187

Grouse

roast	172	1 serving	85	145
roast, with bone	114	1 serving	100	114

Food Category or Brand	Calories /100g	Portion	Size /g	Calories /port
Guinea Fowl				
roast	210	1 serving	85	175
roast, with bone	112	1 serving	100	112
Partridge				
roast, without bone	127	1 serving	100	127
Pheasant				
roast, without bone	134	1 serving	100	134
Pigeon				
boiled	218	1 serving	85	185
boiled, without bone	96	1 serving	120	115
roast, without bone	102	1 serving	120	120
Quail				
roast	321	whole	100	321
Turkey				
roast	195	1 serving	85	165
roast, with bone	117	1 serving	100	117

Branded Poultry Products
Bowyers

chicken roll		each		168
Butterball				
drumstix		each		120
goldencrumb turkey steak		each		135
turkey breast steak		each		100
turkey cheeseburger		each		215
Bernard Matthews				
golden drummer	256			
lamb roast	178			

Food Category or Brand	Calories /100g	Portion	Size /g	Calories /port
mini kiev, cheese & herb		each		42
pork roast	156			
turkey burger, crispy crumb		each		219
turkey fillets	106			
turkey leg roast	132			
turkey thigh mince	127			

Cherry Valley

crispy Peking duck	400			
duckling à l'orange	575			

Iceland

chicken breast steak		each		200
chicken cordon bleu		each		325
chicken finger		each		45
chicken garlic bites		each		50
chicken goujons		each		70
chicken kiev		each		400
turkey nuggets		each		35

Safeway's

chicken breast	106			
chicken breast fillets without skin	148			
chicken roll	133			
cooked chicken breast	111			
frozen skinless chicken breast fillet	106			
honey roast turkey	110			
smoked turkey	109			
turkey rashers	99			
wafer thin honey roast turkey	108			
wafer thin smoked turkey	99			
wafer thin roast chicken	124			

Food Category or Brand	Calories /100g	Portion	Size /g	Calories /port
Sainsbury's				
chicken breast in jelly	98	can		224
economy chicken roll		slice		16
roast chicken (wafer thin)			30	41
smoked turkey (wafer thin)			30	32
St Michael (Marks & Spencer)				
cajun chicken breast	195			
chicken breast	215			
chicken goujons	215			
tangy bbq chicken	230			
Waitrose				
bbq dusted drumsticks	132			
chicken breasts	156			
chicken kiev	199			
chicken wings	230			
farmhouse duck	430			
grouse	144			
lemon & pepper chicken	220			
turkey breast	103			

Nuts

Most nuts contain fat, protein and fibre. Of the more common nuts, only chestnuts contain significant amounts of carbohydrate.

Nuts contain more fat than fatty meat – a Brazil nut is almost two-thirds fat; walnuts, almonds and peanuts are half fat; and hazelnuts and the fleshy part of coconut are one-third fat. Nuts are, therefore, very high in calories. Although amounts vary, about 25 per cent of the fat in nuts is polyunsaturated – in sunflower seeds it is 75 per cent.

Peanuts are the richest in protein at over 25 per cent – weight by weight they contain more protein than a hard cheese like Cheddar. Almonds, Brazils and walnuts, at around 20 per cent, contain weight for weight more protein than egg. However, their protein is of relatively low quality; a nut-based diet would not provide the range and quality of protein required for human life – a fact not always made clear by some advertisements for nuts. Nevertheless, all nut protein can be converted into energy, which is what concerns us here.

Honey roasted and sugar-coated nuts obviously have additional carbohydrates, and therefore more calories.

In the branded section have been included some 'mixed'

assortments, some of which include raisins and other dried fruits.

Food Category or Brand	Calories /100g	Portion	Size /g	Calories /port
Generic Nuts				
Almonds				
kernel	598			
kernel with shells	221			
roasted, salted	607			
Brazils				
kernel	644			
with shells	289			
Cashew nuts				
roasted	559			
Chestnuts				
kernel	172			
with shells	142			
Cobs				
kernel	398			
with shells	143			
Coconut				
fresh	365			
milk (no sugar added)	625			
Macadamias				
roasted, salted	696			
Monkey nuts				
kernel	571			

Food Category or Brand	Calories /100g	Portion	Size /g	Calories /port
Peanuts				
honey roasted	520			
kernel	603			
kernel with shells	416			
roasted, salted	582			
Pecans				
roasted, salted	739			
Pistachios				
with shells	600			
Walnuts				
kernel	549			
with shells	352			

Branded Nuts
KP

	Calories /100g	Portion	Size /g	Calories /port
Brannigans beer nuts	600	1 packet	50	300
honey roasted peanuts	590	1 packet	50	295
large peanuts & raisins	480	1 packet	100	480
mixed nuts & raisins	530	1 packet	50	265
peanuts, raisins & chocolate	480	1 packet	50	240
salt & vinegar peanuts	560	1 packet	50	280

Phileas Fogg

Shanghai nuts	515	1 packet	100	515

Planters

Bombay spiced peanuts	620	1 packet	50	310
dry roasted peanuts	590	1 packet	50	295
hickory smoked peanuts	610	1 packet	50	305
honey peanuts & cashews		1 packet	50	475
honey roasted peanuts	590	1 packet	50	295
salted peanuts	625	1 packet	40	250

Food Category or Brand	Calories /100g	Portion	Size /g	Calories /port
Sainsbury's				
honey cashews & peanuts	392		50	297
luxury fruit & nut mix	355		50	178
luxury nut selection	670		50	335
mixed nuts & raisins	486		50	243
peanuts & raisins	455		50	227
peanuts, raisins & chocolate	469		50	234
salad mixed nuts	628		50	313
salted peanuts	601		50	301
tropical nut mix	447		50	223
St Michael (Marks & Spencer)				
Bombay spice cashews			200	1206
caramelized macadamias			220	2090
cashew			150	929
nuts & fruit			200	1012
peanuts	601			
pistachios			150	903
shelled nuts			200	1314
Sun-Pat				
salted peanuts	615			
Tesco				
blanched peanuts & raisins	411			
cashew nuts	600			
monkey nuts, shelled	571			
natural roast peanuts	585			
peanut kernels	571			
salted mixed nuts	621			
sesame nut crunch	560			
Waitrose				
dry roasted peanuts	617			
roasted salted peanuts	603			

Food Category or Brand	Calories /100g	Portion	Size /g	Calories /port
roasted & salted almonds	637			
salted cashews	615			
salted mixed nuts	582			
salted peanuts	603			
salted pecans	761			
yoghurt coated nuts & raisins	562			

Processed Meats

Sausages, Salamis and Pâtés

Sausages are made from meat, cereal (including bread) and seasonings. The traditional sausage casing is an animal product, but artificial cases also exist. Pork sausages must contain 65 per cent meat, beef sausages 50 per cent. Frankfurters and salami, unless sold canned, must contain 85 per cent meat; the canned versions can go down to 70 per cent meat.

There are no regulations about the amount of fat the 'meat' contains. A regular grilled pork sausage is about 25 per cent fat, 13 per cent protein and slightly less carbohydrate. The rest is water. In a 'low-fat' version the fat element is down to about 14 per cent, the protein proportion moves up to 16 per cent and the carbohydrate 12 per cent. In both cases the fats are either mostly saturated or monounsaturated. Because beef sausages usually have a higher proportion of cereal, weight for weight they contain less fat than pork sausage.

Grilling eliminates between a quarter and a third of the fat. As a result, weight for weight grilled 'regular fat' and 'low-fat' sausages may end up with about the same calorific value. However, the low-fat sausage is still healthier because of the fats lost in its processing.

Frying is not all that different from grilling – almost the same amount of fat is lost.

Salamis and other continental sausages eaten cold often have very high proportions of fat, sometimes in excess of 45 per cent. Carbohydrate is low – less than 2 per cent – protein is 20 per cent and there is usually far less water (under 30 per cent) than in other types of sausage. The fats are solid and therefore very low in polyunsaturates. This explains why there can be 500 kcal in just 100 g of these sausages.

Pâtés and liver sausage are usually between 25 and 30 per cent fat, although certain types of pâté may have up to 45 per cent of fat. Pâtés tend to be moister than salamis, of course, with a water content of over 50 per cent. They contain around 12 to 14 per cent protein and there is almost no carbohydrate. The vast bulk of the fats are saturated. 'Reduced fat' pâtés often show very significant reductions – one manufacturer's regular Brussels pâté is 29 per cent fat, the fat-reduced version only 12 per cent. As a result the calorific value falls from 325 kcal/100 g down to 195 kcal/100 g.

There is no legal distinction between spreads, pastes and pâtés; the cheaper items tend to have a higher proportion of non-meat filler and/or fats as opposed to meat flesh.

Food Category or Brand	Calories /100g	Portion	Size /g	Calories /port
Generic Processed Meats				
beef sausage, fried	287	1 serving	85	245
black sausage	286	1 serving	85	240
frankfurters, canned	220	1 serving	100	220
frankfurters, cooked	303	1 serving	85	255
pork sausage, fried	326	1 serving	85	275
salami, cooked	310	1 serving	85	165
salami, dry	449	1 serving	50	220

Food Category or Brand	Calories /100g	Portion Size /g	Calories /port
Branded Processed Meats			
Bowyers			
garlic sausage	304		
luncheon sausage	282		
Budgens			
garlic sausage	206		
La Rochelle Brussels Pâté	340		
La Rochelle low-fat			
Brussels Pâté	211		
pepperoni	430		
pork & beef sausages	282		
thin-sliced ham	97		
Iceland			
economy thick pork		each	148
economy thick pork & beef		each	115
jumbo pork & beef		each	281
low-fat thick pork		each	93
premium pork		each	198
thick beef		each	144
thick pork		each	144
thick pork & beef		each	150
thick pork & herbs		each	135
thin pork		each	72
thin pork & beef		each	75
Mattesons			
black pudding	354		
bratwurst	336		
frankfurters	354		
garlic German	248		
ham	142		
liver	265		

Food Category or Brand	Calories /100g	Portion	Size /g	Calories /port
Safeway				
cubed pork – super trim	122			
diced braising steak	129			
diced stewing steak	129			
lean pork mince	121			
pork escalopes – super trim	120			
sliced braising steak – super trim	129			
thick pork sausages	209			
Sainsbury's				
chorizo		each		91
extra lean sausages		each		88
frankfurters		each		114
hot dogs		each		68
Lincolnshire sausages		each		155
pastrami		slice		14
pepperoni		serving	30	95
pork		each		132
St Michael (Marks & Spencer)				
black pudding		each	38	340
butchers sausages	310			
chorizo sausage	230			
Cumberland sausages	270			
leek and Caerphilly sausage	250			
Lincolnshire sausage	265			
pork sausage	350			
Toulouse sausage	215			
Waitrose				
beef Napolitana sausage	237			
cajun pork sausage	309			
chambelle salami	407			
chicken liver pâté	251			

Food Category or Brand	Calories /100g	Portion	Size /g	Calories /port
Cumberland sausage	268			
duck & pork pâté	228			
French salami	438			
pastrami	120			
pork & beef sausages	259			
pork & leek sausage	303			
pork chipolatas	290			
Toulouse pork sausage	266			

Walls

light & lean country	198			
light & lean premium	178			
Lincolnshire		each		113
pork & beef	282			

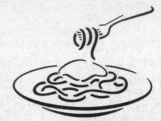

Ready-made Meals

What are called here 'ready-made meals' are those substantial dishes you can buy at the supermarket, sold either frozen or chilled, which need simple heating. In some cases the identical dish is sold both chilled (for eating almost immediately) and frozen (for longer-term storage). In the listings we have grouped together canned meals; fresh, frozen and chilled meals; pies and pastries; and lunch/snack bowls and pot meals.

Increasingly the range is including a number of ethnic dishes, prepared with an increasing amount of authenticity. See also the **Meat and Poultry, Rice, Pasta and Pizza**, and **Vegetarian Dishes** sections.

Dishes with identical names but different brand labels may be made from very different recipes. Although it is an open secret that some well-known food manufacturers make 'own-brand' products for rival supermarkets as well as selling goods under their own name, that does not mean that they will use the same recipes; indeed, every one of the UK's main supermarket chains imposes its own very high standards.

It is with ready-made dishes that 'guessing calories by looking' becomes most difficult. Dishes based on pies, flans, pasta and rice will be relatively high in carbohydrates. In the case of pies and flans – and Indian samosas – the pastry will also contain fats.

Breaded dishes will also have plenty of carbohydrates, there will be fat in the binder, and if the breaded dish is then fried as opposed to grilled, fat will be absorbed during the cooking process. Pancake-based dishes are similar. Rice-based dishes will have the lowest amount of fats.

Although meat dishes should be relatively high in protein, there may be considerable amounts of fat not only in sausage- and mince-based dishes, but also in pies, pasties and stews.

Many sauces are based on cream or cheese – these will add considerably to the fat content and the fat itself will be low in polyunsaturates. Some tomato sauces contain surprising amounts of sugar.

Neither freezing nor canning has any direct effect on the calorific value of dishes; other nutritional qualities, however, notably vitamins, may be lost.

Microwaving and grilling cooking methods are preferable to frying. However, as a general health warning, particular care should be taken with microwaving chilled dishes – uneven cooking can result in cold spots where food has been inadequately heated and may therefore be unsafe.

Food Category or Brand	Calories /100g	Portion	Size /g	Calories /port
Canned Meals				
Baxters				
boeuf bourguignon	98			
coq au vin	77			

Food Category or Brand	Calories /100g	Portion	Size /g	Calories /port
Co-op				
beef casserole	73			
chilli con carne	159			
Irish stew	80			
steak & kidney pie	314			
vegetable curry	84			
Fray Bentos				
beef curry	91			
chicken & mushroom pie	145			
minced beef & onion pie	215			
steak & ale pie	216			
steak & kidney pie	170			
Heinz				
baked beans with chicken nuggets	104			
baked beans & pork sausages	110			
curried beans	113			
Sainsbury's				
beef casserole		can		364
chicken curry		can		512
chicken in white wine sauce		can		706
chilli con carne		can		450

Fresh, Frozen & Chilled Meals

Asda

Food Category or Brand	Calories /100g	Portion	Size /g	Calories /port
beef & vegetable Yorkshire	64			
beef canneloni	98			
beef curry with rice	126			
beef Madras	168			
chicken & broccoli pasta bake	186			
chicken balti	133			
chicken casserole with mash	74			

Food Category or Brand	Calories /100g	Portion Size /g		Calories /port
Lancashire hot pot	68			
lasagne	126			
macaroni cheese	163			
meatballs & pasta	132			
pork szechuan Chinese	132			
roasted vegetable potato melt	112			
spaghetti Bolognaise with pasta	96			
spicy tuna & pasta	95			
spinach & ricotta cannelloni	135			
sweet & sour chicken with rice	94			
tagliatelle carbonara	112			
tuna & pasta bake	120			
vegetable hotpot	96			

Birds Eye Wall's

Food Category or Brand	Calories /100g	Portion Size /g		Calories /port
beef stew with dumplings		serving		320
chicken & vegetable pie		pie		159
chilli con carne		pack		285
chicken supreme with rice		pack		375
creamy mustard chicken with rice		serving		375
fettucini Bolognese		serving		500
macaroni cheese		meal		285
Mediterranean chicken with sun-dried tomatoes		serving		450
roast dinners		dinner		340
spicy beef noodles		serving		500
sweet & sour chicken & rice		pack		350
various curries with rice		serving		375
vegetable curry with rice		pack		350

HEALTHY OPTIONS

Food Category or Brand	Calories /100g	Portion Size /g		Calories /port
beef pasta bolognese		serving		350
chicken korma & rice		serving		350
chicken tikka masala dinner		serving		368
glazed chicken dinner		serving		368

Food Category or Brand	Calories /100g	Portion	Size /g	Calories /port
lasagne		serving		375
roast vegetable and tomato pasta		serving		350

Co-op
beef stew & dumplings	119			
cauliflower cheese	135			
chicken korma	123			
chicken tikka masala with pilau rice	205			
chilli con carne & rice	113			
cottage pie	101			
cowboys dinner	112			
ranch time lunch	93			
rogan josh	123			
sausage casserole	147			
toad in the hole	222			

Ross Young's
Caribbean chicken	74			
Chinese special rice	116			
cod crumble	179			
deep dish lasagne	151			
fish mornay	137			
Japanese beef Oriental	65			
Lancashire hot pot	102			
Ocean Classic's paella	94			
Ocean Classic's seafood crumble	197			
ocean pie	117			

Safeway
bangers, beans & mash	151			
basmati & wild rice pilaff	119			
beef curry with rice	116			
beef stew & dumpling	98			

Food Category or Brand	Calories /100g	Portion	Size /g	Calories /port
chicken & broccoli pasta bake	85			
chicken chow mein	101			
chicken korma with rice	167			
chicken tikka masala with rice	133			
chilli con carne with rice	113			
herb & garlic satay	139			
lamb samosa	247			
Lancashire hot pot	100			
onion bhaji	216			
sweet & sour chicken with rice	99			

Sainsbury's

Food Category or Brand	Calories /100g	Portion	Size /g	Calories /port
Bombay potato		pack		200
Cantonese chicken with mushrooms		pack		264
Cantonese sweet & sour chicken with rice		pack		471
chicken & cashew nuts with rice		pack		384
chicken biryani		pack		544
chicken tikka massala		pack		650
Cumberland pie		pack		664
fisherman's pie		pack		336
lamb rogan josh		pack		522
Lancashire hot pot		pack		534
moussaka		pack		810
onion bhaji		each		84
shepherds pie		pack		662
tandoori chicken sizzler		pack		404

St Michael (Marks & Spencer)

Food Category or Brand	Calories /100g	Portion	Size /g	Calories /port
Angus minced beef pie	280			
beef escalopes in gravy	125			
chicken and bacon lattice	275			
chicken and cashew nuts	95			
chicken casserole	115			

Food Category or Brand	Calories /100g	Portion	Size /g	Calories /port
chicken jalfrezi	150			
chicken risotto	125			
chicken satay	210			
chicken tikka	165			
chicken/mushroom/potato	130			
lamb casserole	95			
lamb rogan josh	100			
lasagne	160			
meatballs in gravy	165			
plaice Florentine	120			
roast beef meal	130			
roast duck and plum sauce	175			
rump of lamb	175			
salmon and noodle parcels	120			
salmon and spinach risotto	140			
salmon fishcakes	195			
sausage and potato casserole	95			
steak and ale	111			
steak carbonade	100			
steak meal	85			
sweet & sour chicken	100			
Thai style fishcakes	95			

Waitrose

bacon, onion, watercress flan	323			
beef stroganoff	117			
chicken biryani	183			
chicken chasseur	87			
chicken lasagne	108			
crispy Peking duck	207			
king prawn masala	120			
moussaka	160			
salmon & prawn tagliatelle	103			
smoked salmon souffle	176			
sweet & sour pork	293			
Thai green chicken curry	193			

Food Category or Brand	Calories /100g	Portion	Size /g	Calories /port
Weight Watchers from Heinz				
beef lasagne		pack	295	288
chicken korma with rice		pack	290	282
chicken Mexicana with rice		pack	320	286
vegetable hot-pot		pack	335	230
vegetable lasagne		pack	320	286
Pies and Pastries				
Birds Eye Wall's				
chicken pie	280			
minced beef & onion pie	280			
steak & kidney pie	279			
Boots				
cheese & onion rolls		pack		335
chicken, sweetcorn & mushroom pasty		pack		286
chicken, vegetable & cheese pasty		pack		273
ratatouille cheese topped pie		pack		277
traditional Cornish pasty		pack		466
Co-op				
chicken satay flan	195			
corned beef flan	253			
deep-filled chicken & vegetable pie	218			
deep-filled quorn & mushroom pie	248			
flan quorn & leek	242			
meat & potato pie	275			
pork pie	390			
potato, cheese & onion pasty	267			
quiche/egg, cheese & onion flan	213			

Food Category or Brand	Calories /100g	Portion	Size /g	Calories /port
sausage rolls (5)	413			
wholemeal Provençale quiche	232			
vegetable pasty	293			
Ross Young				
Cornish pasties	228			
family chicken & vegetable	232			
family steak & kidney	270			
minced beef & onion	276			
minced beef & onion pasties	259			
Sainsbury's				
chicken & mushroom slice		each		450
chicken & vegetable pie		each		385
chicken, mushroom & broccoli				
roll		each		978
Cornish pasty		each		401
deep filled steak pie		each		1316
minced beef and onion pie		each		1182
pork sausage rolls		each		231
salmon & broccoli flan		each		880
steak & kidney pie		each		349
Waitrose				
chicken & broccoli	284			
Cornish pasty	266			
minced beef & onion	274			
pork, cheese & pickle	418			
roast chicken, mushroom				
& bacon	256			
savoury cod	148			
steak & kidney	248			

Food Category or Brand	Calories /100g	Portion	Size /g	Calories /port
Lunch/Snack Bowls and Pot Meals				
Golden Wonder				
POT MASH				
spicy curry	352	pot		289
sausage & tomato	354	pot		301
POT NOODLE				
beef & tomato	408	pot		367
chicken & mushroom	403	pot		359
spicy curry	426	pot		380
chow mein	424	pot		369
sweet & sour	435	pot		375
nice & spicy	424	pot		369
POT RICE				
chicken curry	346	pot		257
chicken & sweetcorn	352	pot		240
Heinz				
LUNCHBOWL				
beef curry with rice	84			
chicken curry with rice	105			
country vegetable casserole	57			
lamb & vegetable casserole	81			
spaghetti bolognese	109			
MICROWAVE LUNCHBOX				
chicken curry with rice	105		215	227
spaghetti bolognese	109		215	257

Rice, Pasta and Pizza

Rice

Rice is mostly carbohydrate in the form of starch; brown rice has more protein than white since only the outer husk of the plant has been removed. There are also very small quantities of oil in rice, about half of which is polyunsaturated.

Raw white rice is 11 per cent water; by the time it has been cooked the proportion of water is between 65 and 70 per cent. Differences in the calorific value of various types of dried rice – basmati, pilau, Italian – usually depend on the amount of moisture in the grain. The different types of grain also absorb water in the cooking process to varying extents, and this too can result in apparently anomalous calorific values.

Rice is usually boiled but is also fried; however, in most frying processes only small amounts of oil are absorbed. For the health-conscious it is better to fry in oils than in solid fats; in Indian cooking *ghee* – clarified butter – is used. Chinese fried rice may also contain egg – this will then increase the amounts of fat and cholesterol; however the overall dish would still be categorized as low in fats.

Prepared rice dishes – or side-dishes – containing vegetables will have, weight for weight, lower energy values than portions of rice alone. Also see the sections on **Ethnic Foods** and **Ready-made Meals**.

Pasta

Basic pasta is made from milled durum wheat and water, which is made into a dough and then rolled, shaped and cut. It is now widely sold 'fresh' as well as in the traditional dried form. This means that nutritional data as it appears on a pack may be for cooked pasta – when it will have absorbed large quantities of water – for uncooked fresh, or uncooked dry. Raw 'dried' pasta still has a water content of 9 or 10 per cent; by the time it is cooked the water content is above 70 per cent. A fresh pasta has a moisture content of about 30 per cent.

In a dry pasta most of the energy is in the form of carbohydrate – as starch – and will be about 75 per cent of the total content. Protein will be about 12 per cent and fat 2 per cent. Some pasta – tagliatelle, for example – is made with egg, the main effect being to increase the fat content to 8–10 per cent.

A simple pasta sauce of tomatoes and minced meat will have a much lower calorific value than one containing eggs or olive oil, or where the dish has been liberally sprinkled with Parmesan cheese (see the section on **Dairy Products**).

One manufacturer's canned spaghetti bolognese may be quite different from another's, and again one brand of chilled or frozen lasagne may have a very different calorific value than another. Even 'tomato sauce' can vary considerably, depending on the amount of sugar used in it. The table below will give you an idea of the range.

We have also included some pasta sauces. A few pasta-related dishes also appear in the **Ready-made Meals** section.

Pizza

Pizza dough is principally carbohydrate in the form of starch. The classic pizza covering is tomato sauce and cheese – the margharita – plus various possible additions. A typical pizza of this type is just over 50 per cent water, 25 per cent carbohydrate (of which 2 to 3 per cent will be sugars), 9 per cent protein and 12 per cent fat. Just under half the fat will be saturated and will come mostly from the cheese.

Deep-pan and 'French bread' pizzas have, weight for weight, lower energy values, higher proportions of carbohydrate and lower proportions of fats than more traditional thin-crust pizzas.

The pizzas listed are 'ready-made' dishes that you heat/cook yourself. Some are deep-frozen (listed as 'frozen' in this table), others will be found in your supermarket's chill cabinet. You can use the data given here as the basis for estimating the calorie content of pizzas you make yourself from basic ingredients or those you eat in restaurants.

Information about favourite products from the popular pizza restaurant chains can be found in the **Fast Foods** section, while information about other Italian specialities appear in the **Ethnic Foods** section.

Food Category or Brand	Calories /100g	Portion	Size /g	Calories /port
Generic Rice				
Basmati				
boiled	225			
raw	357			

Food Category or Brand	Calories /100g	Portion Size /g	Calories /port
Brown & Wild			
raw	325		
Caribbean			
cooked	125		
raw	500		
Easy-cook			
cooked	138		
Pilau (Pilaff)			
boiled	220		
raw	350		
Pudding rice			
cooked	95		
Quick-cook			
cooked	125		
Quinoa			
raw	346		
Risotto			
cooked	180		
White, polished			
boiled	100		
Wholegrain brown			
cooked	160		

Food Category or Brand	Calories /100g	Portion	Size /g	Calories /port
Branded Rice				
Batchelors Savoury				
beef		per packet		435
chicken		per packet		440
Chinese chicken, fried		per packet		615
Chinese special, fried		per packet		580
Chinese sweet & sour		per packet		640
golden or mushroom		per packet		445
hot Indian		per packet		665
Indian special, fried		per packet		660
mild curry		per packet		425
Mediterranean		per packet		540
tandoori special, fried		per packet		635
wholegrain mixed vegetable		per packet		425
Co-op Savoury				
beef or mushroom		per packet		435
chicken curry		per packet		430
mixed vegetable		per packet		425
Ross				
Chinese special	121	1 serving	120	145
stir-fry rice mix	71	1 serving	120	85
Safeway				
BOIL IN THE BAG				
basmati rice	350			
brown rice	347			
white rice	350			
Sainsbury's				
American wholegrain brown rice			50	169
easy cook American rice			50	179

Food Category or Brand	Calories /100g	Portion	Size /g	Calories /port
St Michael (Marks & Spencer)				
Basmati rice	339			
Italian risotto rice	336			
long grain & wild rice	339			
long grain rice	337			
Thai rice	342			
Tesco				
mild curry rice, raw	314			
mild curry rice, cooked	106			
mixed vegetable rice, raw	316			
mixed vegetable rice, cooked	111			
Tilda				
easy cook Basmati long-grain, raw	335			
Basmati & wild rice	330			
Basmati rice	330			
Uncle Ben's				
aromatic blend rice	344			
basmati rice	343			
long grain rice	347			
pilau rice	335			
supreme basmati rice	350			
Thai fragrant rice	346			
Thai imperial rice	346			
veetee rice	330			
wholegrain rice	340			
Waitrose				
basmati rice	350			
boil in a bag brown rice	345			
easy cook rice	370			
long grain brown rice	345			

Food Category or Brand	Calories /100g	Portion	Size /g	Calories /port
long grain rice	347			
pudding rice	318			

Generic Dried Pasta
macaroni	360	1 serving	75	270
noodles	364	1 serving	75	273
spaghetti	365	1 serving	75	274
spirals, wholewheat	275	1 serving	75	206
twists	344	1 serving	75	258

Generic Fresh Pasta
capelliti	156	1 serving	75	117
ravioli	318	1 serving	75	239
tagliatelle	156	1 serving	75	117
tortelloni, five-cheese	304	1 serving	75	228

Branded Pasta
Buitoni
conchiglie pasta	362			
eliche pasta	362			
farfelle pasta	362			
gnocchi pasta	362			
penne rigate pasta	362			

Co-op
spaghetti in tomato sauce	58	1 can	410	240
wholewheat spaghetti in tomato sauce	58	1 can	410	240

Crosse & Blackwell
Alphabetti spaghetti		1 can	425	255
Fred Bear beans & pasta		1 can	440	360
higher-fibre spaghetti		1 can	425	255
spaghetti rings		1 can	213	140
straight spaghetti		1 can	213	140

Food Category or Brand	Calories /100g	Portion	Size /g	Calories /port
wholewheat spaghetti		1 can	213	130
Findus				
cannelloni	119	1 serving	200	238
lasagne	121	1 serving	242	292
Heinz				
macaroni cheese		1 can	210	205
ravioli in tomato sauce	74	1 can	215	165
spaghetti hoops		1 can	215	135
spaghetti in tomato sauce	65	1 can	215	135
Weight Watchers spaghetti		1 can	215	115
Iceland				
boiled pasta mix	57			
mixed vegetables with pasta spirals	68			
KP				
bolognaise quick lunch		1 tub		150
Napolina				
ravioli in tomato & beef sauce		1 can	411	370
ravioli in tomato sauce		1 can	411	350
Ross				
lasagne	120			
macaroni cheese	110			
Safeway				
cappelletti with basil pesto	315			
cappelletti with chicken & smoked ham	264			
chonchigliell	349			
ditale rigato	349			

Food Category or Brand	Calories /100g	Portion	Size /g	Calories /port
farfilline	349			
panzotti with smoked salmon	272			
tagliatelle with garlic & herbs	289			
tortelloni with five cheeses	309			
tortelloni with garlic & herbs	273			
tortelloni with cheese & sundried tomatoes	301			

Sainsbury's

garlic & herb tortelloni		pack		776
gnocchi		pack		656
lasagne		serving		317
lasagne di spinaci		serving		475
raviolini		serving		394
spinach & ricotta tortelloni		pack		742
tagliatelle		pack		682

St Michael (Marks & Spencer)

fiorelli	372			
fusilli	358			
pappardelle	365			
penne	355			
spaghetti	351			
tagliatelle	366			

Waitrose

farfalle	354			
fusilli	547			
gnocchi	354			
pasta quills	354			
stelline	354			
tagliatelle nests	354			

Food Category or Brand	Calories /100g	Portion	Size /g	Calories /port
Pasta sauces				
Ragu				
broccoli & white wine	62	jar		273
courgette & aubergine	50	jar		220
parmesan style	90	jar		396
red wine & herbs	84	jar		370
traditional	79	jar		348
Safeway				
amatriciana	70			
bolognese	73			
carbonara	193			
creamy mushroom	114			
creamy tomato & olive	88			
four cheese	223			
napoletana	37			
pepper & basil	47			
tomato with mushrooms	67			
tomato with onions & garlic	67			
tomato with pepper	68			
traditional pasta sauce	67			
Sainsbury's				
carbonara		pot		345
classic pasta sauce (jar)		pot		92
florentina		pot		172
napoletana		pot		83
St Michael (Marks & Spencer)				
bolognaise	85			
green pesto	411			
olive pasta sauce	335			
roasted Italian vegetable	232			
roasted red pepper	55			
romana	90			

Food Category or Brand	Calories /100g	Portion	Size /g	Calories /port
spicy pepper sauce	175			
spicy sausage sauce	65			
spinach/ricotta	245			
tomato & herb	50			
tomato & mascarpone	80			
tomato & pesto	70			

Waitrose

crushed Italian tomatoes & herbs	30			
crushed sundried tomatoes	514			
Italian funghi sauce	75			
napoletana sauce	66			
pasta sauce garlic	58			
pesto sauce in olive oil	373			

Branded Pizza

Findus

CRISPY BASE

cheese & tomato	208			
ham	168			

FRENCH BREAD

bacon, peppers & mushroom	192			
Italian sausage	183			
savoury barbecue	223			
tomato & cheese	228			

FROZEN

barbecue beef		1 pizza		400
ham & pineapple	188	1 pizza	170	320

Iceland

cheese & tomato		1 pizza		234
ham & mushroom		1 pizza		225

Food Category or Brand	Calories /100g	Portion	Size /g	Calories /port
McVitie's				
pizza pie		1 pizza		440
Ross				
cheese & onion	210	1 pizza		190
crispy bacon	250	1 pizza		230
French bread pizza	270	1 pizza		380
ham, mushroom & cheese	220	1 pizza		200
tomato & cheese	220	1 pizza		200
wholemeal tomato & cheese	237	1 pizza		210
Sainsbury's				
bacon & mushroom		each		848
garlic & mushroom		each		746
ham & pineapple		each		842
quattro formaggi		each		764
Waitrose				
bacon & mushroom	216			
Italian proscuitto	226			
Italiane 5 cheese	220			
spicy sausage	222			
spinach & broccoli	207			
thin & crispy cheese & tomato	186			
tomato & cheese	212			

Sandwiches

Sandwiches are often thought of as snacks, but that doesn't mean they're necessarily low in calories. Those that contain mayonnaise or other oil- or dairy-rich sauces (see **Dairy Products** and **Fats and Oils**) may be very high-calorie indeed.

The sandwiches listed here are the types sold chilled and sealed in clear plastic cases. The life of this type of sandwich is prolonged by the use of inert gases sealed into the package, which keep oxygen out and thereby keep the sandwich fresher longer.

Unwrapped sandwiches sold in other outlets will have similar calorific values, though in general the sealed sandwiches tend to have more substantial fillings.

Also see the section on **Bread**.

Food Category or Brand	Calories /100g	Portion	Size /g	Calories /port
Branded Sandwiches				
Asda				
BLT	236			
brie & bacon	333			
cheese & coleslaw	305			

Food Category or Brand	Calories /100g	Portion	Size /g	Calories /port
cheese & tomato	305			
chicken & bacon	277			
chicken & sweetcorn	247			
chicken tikka	170			
corned beef & onion	328			
egg salad	175			
ham & turkey tower	206			
ploughmans	256			
prawn & egg	228			
prawn mayonnaise	220			
red salmon & cucumber	191			
roast beef & onion	233			
seafood cocktail	256			
tuna & cucumber	192			

Boots Shapers

FLATBREADS

chicken & blackbean	122	pack		250
chicken caesar	179	pack		302
chicken tikka	167	pack		295
Chinese pork	147	pack		268
cottage cheese	186	pack		310
fajita	138	pack		275
feta cheese	172	pack		287
Italian chicken	191	pack		320
Italian salad	144	pack		294
Moroccan chicken	176	pack		271
oriental chicken & mango	161	pack		289
spicy Mexican	156	pack		297

REGULAR SANDWICHES

BLT	192	pack		328
cheese and Branston	207	pack		341
cheese and onion Swedish	209	pack		266
cheese salad	185	pack		308

Food Category or Brand	Calories /100g	Portion	Size /g	Calories /port
cheese tomato & spring onion	192	pack		344
chick/prawn/blt	182	pack		403
chicken & bacon	180	pack		322
chicken tikka	159	pack		327
egg mayo & cress	189	pack		305
egg mayo & tomato	172	pack		340
egg salad	165	pack		304
ham & cheese Swedish	205	pack		258
ham & double Gloucester	165	pack		324
ham soft cheese pineapple	176	pack		295
lemon chicken	183	pack		315
Louisiana bagel	191	pack		312
oriental chicken triple	185	pack		398
prawn cocktail salad	177	pack		396
prawn mayo triple	195	pack		433
roast chicken	177	pack		288
roast chicken salad	147	pack		284
salmon & cucumber	184	pack		327
salmon & soft cheese bagel	218	pack		345
simply salad	139	pack		301
tomato, parmesan & rocket	85	pack		303
tuna & cucumber	180	pack		323
tuna & lemon mayo	154	pack		318
tuna melt swedish	158	pack		258
tuna pepper & sweetcorn	169	pack		306
turkey ham & coleslaw	146	pack		337
vegetarian triple	175	pack		421
Safeway				
bacon, lettuce & tomato		pack		406
cheese & celery		pack		400
cheese & pickle		pack		432
chicken tikka		pack		446
Chinese chicken		pack		292
egg mayonnaise		pack		372

Food Category or Brand	Calories /100g	Portion	Size /g	Calories /port
Ploughman's pack		pack		599
prawn mayonnaise		pack		565
roast chicken & salad		pack		396
tuna & cucumber		pack		392
ROLLS				
Flamed chicken		pack		361
Ploughman's Salad		pack		522
Somerset camembert with apple & mayonnaise		pack		470
REDUCED CALORIE				
egg salad		pack		259
lemon chicken		pack		277
roast chicken with yoghurt & cream		pack		280
smoked turkey salad		pack		276
HEALTHY CHOICE RANGE				
bacon, lettuce & tomato		pack		297
egg mayonnaise and cress		pack		291
prawn & mayonnaise		pack		317
roast chicken with salad		pack		309
tuna & cucumber		pack		268
TRIPLE PACKS				
BLT, egg & bacon, sausage with brown sauce		pack		551
cheese & celery, roast chicken & salad, tuna & cucumber		pack		582
chicken		pack		573

egg mayonnaise & cress,
    cheese & coleslaw, prawn
    mayonnaise
		pack		647

honey roast ham salad		pack		211

Food Category or Brand	Calories /100g	Portion	Size /g	Calories /port
Sainsbury's				
chargrilled chicken		pack		374
cheddar & pickle		pack		396
chicken & bacon		pack		511
deep filled, cheese & tomato		pack		541
deep filled, chicken & ham		pack		460
deep filled, egg & tomato		pack		489
ham & Edam		pack		486
hummus, carrot & salad		pack		358
Lincolnshire pork sausage		pack		428
mature cheddar & onion		pack		782
mixed salad		pack		348
mozzarella & tomato		pack		420
ploughman's		pack		358
prawn & mayo		pack		460
Thai chicken		pack		434
REDUCED CALORIE				
chicken & coleslaw		pack		332
tuna & cucumber		pack		268
turkey		pack		256
TRIPLES				
BLT, sausage & mustard, egg & bacon		pack		718
chicken tikka, Thai chicken, chicken korma		pack		588
prawn mayo, salmon & cucumber tuna & mayo		pack		516
smoked ham, egg & cress, cheddar & tomato		pack		587
ROLLS				
cheese ploughman's		roll		541
egg florentine		bloomer		458

Food Category or Brand	Calories /100g	Portion	Size /g	Calories /port
egg salad		roll		428
ham & cheese		roll		461
prawn salad		roll		415

St Michael (Marks & Spencer)

BLT	321
bacon/chicken/avocado	229
beef/onion	231
cheese & onion	220
chicken coleslaw	211
egg & cress	195
ham cheese pickle	233
prawn & mayo	244
roast chicken	203

ROLLS

chicken salad	238
ham & egg	240
prawn & egg	265
spicy prawn	220

BAGUETTE

ham & cheese	285
tuna & mayo	270

Waitrose

bacon triple pack	252
cheese & coleslaw	234
cheese & pickle	242
chicken salad	224
ham & tomato	207
prawn, lemon mayo	239
reduced fat chicken	168
reduced fat prawn & mayo	210
reduced fat tuna & celery	174

Soups

Fairly obviously, soups are mostly water. Their energy component comes from carbohydrate (as starch).

Meat-based soups may contain small amounts of fat. The real trap lies in thickened soups. Potato-based thickening – as in parmentiers – adds only carbohydrate; the same is true of cornflower and ground pulses as additives – but cream and eggs will add fats and protein.

The manufacturers' figures for powdered soups are usually for the powder itself rather than the cooked (and very much diluted) soup. The main difference between a cup soup and a conventional packet soup is cooking time.

Food Category or Brand	Calories /100g	Portion Size /g	Calories /port
Canned Soups			
Asda			
chicken	39		
cream of celery	45		
cream of tomato	74		
minestrone	26		
tomato	52		
vegetable	27		

Food Category or Brand	Calories /100g	Portion	Size /g	Calories /port
Baxters				
SPECIAL OCCASION/LUXURY RANGE				
beef consommé	16			
cream of courgette	62			
cream of salmon	58			
Cullen Skink	85			
lobster bisque	53			
mushroom pottage	73			
spicy Thai chicken	67			
TRADITIONAL RANGE				
chicken broth	32			
chicken noodle	36			
cock-a-leekie	22			
cream of tomato	69			
French onion	21			
lentil & bacon	45			
minestrone	34			
pea & ham	75			
royal game	28			
Scotch broth	39			
VEGETARIAN SOUPS				
carrot & butter bean	47			
country garden	28			
potato & leek	36			
spicy parsnip	49			
tomato & orange	40			
Campbells				
CONDENSED STANDARD				
cream of chicken	50			
cream of mushroom	52			
cream of tomato	66			
cream of onion	42			

Food Category or Brand	Calories /100g	Portion	Size /g	Calories /port
oxtail	40			
Scotch broth	40			
vegetable	32			
CONDENSED SPECIAL CHOICE				
chicken & mushroom	44			
cream of asparagus	45			
ham & cheese	57			
Italian tomato & basil	68			
mushroom & garlic	52			
GRANNY SOUPS				
lentil & bacon	53			
pea & ham	62			
potato & leek	38			
tomato	56			
Heinz				
beef	45			
chicken & mushroom	51			
cream of asparagus	52			
cream of mushroom	54			
cream of tomato	72			
minestrone	31			
BIG SOUP				
beef & vegetable	39			
chicken & vegetable	39			
thick country veg & ham	46			
FARMHOUSE				
beef & vegetable	39			
potato & leek	35			
Scotch broth	44			

Food Category or Brand	Calories /100g	Portion /g	Size /port	Calories
WHOLESOUP				
country vegetable	51			
tomato & lentil	54			
winter vegetable	47			

Sainsbury's

celery			can	232
chicken noodle			can	108
cream of chicken			can	278
cream of mushroom			can	248
cream of tomato			can	310
economy tomato			can	276
extra thick vegetable			can	238
lentil with bacon			can	244
minestrone			can	196
mulligatawny			can	174
oxtail			can	138
pea & ham			can	274
potato & leek			can	238
vegetable & beef			can	276

Weight Watchers from Heinz

celery				64
chicken noodle				58
lentil & carrot				76
minestrone				53
Wholesome Soup, curried vegetable				96

Fresh Soups
New Covent Garden

broccoli & stilton cheese soup	53	½ carton	284	151
carrot and coriander soup	50	½ carton	284	142
cream of chicken with lemon & tarragon soup	59	½ carton	284	168
leek and potato soup	37	½ carton	284	105

Food Category or Brand	Calories /100g	Portion /g	Size /port	Calories
lentil & tomato with cumin				
& coriander soup	57	½ carton	284	162
minestrone soup	33	½ carton	284	94
plum tomato soup	40	½ carton	284	114
Sicilian tomato soup	34	½ carton	284	97
spinach with nutmeg soup	43	½ carton	284	122
Thai spinach soup	61	½ carton	284	173
Tuscan bean soup	47	½ carton	284	133
wild mushroom soup	44	½ carton	284	125

Safeway

Food Category or Brand	Calories /100g	Portion /g	Size /port	Calories
broccoli & cheddar	73			
carrot & orange	48			
country vegetable soup	56			
creamy mushroom	67			
Italian style tomato	52			
mixed bean soup	59			
spicy carrot with parsnip &				
apple	54			

Sainsbury's

Food Category or Brand	Calories /100g	Portion /g	Size /port	Calories
broccoli & stilton			bottle	274
carrot & coriander			bottle	234
chicken & sweetcorn			bottle	160
cream of chicken			bottle	300
tomato & basil			bottle	166
wild mushroom			bottle	202

St Michael (Marks & Spencer)

Food Category or Brand	Calories /100g	Portion /g	Size /port	Calories
carrot & parsnip	32			
country vegetable	57			
creamy chicken	110			
lentil & bacon	60			
minestrone	46			
pea & ham	60			
tomato & herb	70			

Food Category or Brand	Calories /100g	Portion /g	Size /port	Calories
tomato & lentil	45			
winter vegetable	40			

Waitrose
chicken & sweetcorn	55			
cream of asparagus	57			
cream of tomato	67			
French onion	26			
lentil & bacon	53			
minestrone	51			
oxtail soup	37			
pea & ham	55			
Tuscan bean	47			
vegetable soup	40			

Packet Soups
Batchelors Cup Soups
chicken & mushroom	221	1 packet		62
golden vegetable	250	1 packet		70
minestrone (with croutons)	250	1 packet		70
onion	393	1 packet		110
thick mushroom	386	1 packet		108
tomato	296	1 packet		83
vegetable & beef	307	1 packet		86

Holland & Barrett
soup mixes	285	1 packet		81

Knorr
chicken & leek	338	1 packet		233
chicken noodle	347	1 packet		187
Cornish seafood	374	1 packet		278
lentil	314	1 packet		301
minestrone	312	1 packet		243
oxtail	327	1 packet		250

Food Category or Brand	Calories /100g	Portion /g	Size /port	Calories
pea with ham	327	1 packet		250
spring vegetable	280	1 packet		106
sweetcorn	368	1 packet		328
thick vegetable	310	1 packet		242

Sainsbury's

SOUP IN A CUP

chicken			sachet	84
farmhouse vegetable			sachet	75
reduced calorie farmhouse vegetable			sachet	38
reduced calorie minestrone			sachet	55

'SPECIALS' RANGE

chicken & mushroom			sachet	105
chicken & vegetable			sachet	116
harvest vegetable			sachet	97
minestrone			sachet	84
tomato			sachet	112

Sugar, Syrups, Confectionery and Cereal Bars

Confectionery

Chocolate is approximately 30 per cent fat and 60 per cent carbohydrate. It has very little water or protein. The main fat component is saturated fat; nearly all of the carbohydrate is sugars rather than starch.

There is hardly any difference in the calorific value of the various sorts of chocolate – brown, dark brown, white, flavoured. Most 'filled' chocolate bars have, weight for weight, a lower calorific value than solid chocolate. Milk chocolate is rather fattier than plain and also contains cholesterol.

Most 'sweets' are almost pure carbohydrate, chiefly complex sugars. They provide instant energy – hence the use of glucose tablets by athletes and those with long work schedules – but are otherwise of no nutritional value.

Cereal Bars

Despite their boast of 100 per cent natural ingredients and the undoubted benefits of the dietary fibre they contain – up to 20 per cent in some cases – cereal bars are not especially good for you. Typical calorific values are 400 to 500 kcal/100 g, of which nearly half will be carbohydrate. Half of this carbohydrate is sugar. This means that a typical 100 g bar contains 25 g of sugar – five teaspoons-full!

Protein is likely to be less than 10 per cent. Oil, usually mostly unsaturated, will be just under 20 per cent. The 'chewy' type of bar will usually have a higher proportion of fats.

Chocolate-coated bars will have additional saturated fats and sugar. Carob coating adds over 100 kcal/100 g to the bar; yoghurt coating adds 130 kcal/100 g.

If you are on a calorie-controlled diet with the aim of losing weight rather than gaining it, do yourself a favour and try to avoid everything listed in this section.

Food Category or Brand	Calories /100g	Portion	Size /g	Calories /port
Sugar				
demerara	394			
white	394			
Syrups				
corn	289			
maple	251			
golden	297			
Generic Chocolate				
milk	588			
plain	544			
Branded Chocolate				
Aero		1 bar		250
Applause		1 bar		220
Bounty, milk		1 bar		275
Bounty, plain		1 bar		270

Food Category or Brand	Calories /100g	Portion	Size /g	Calories /port
Crunchie		1 bar		195
Curly Wurly		1 bar		130
Dairy Milk (Cadbury's)		1 bar		255
Dime		1 bar		160
Flake		1 bar		170
Galaxy		1 bar		273
Kit Kat		1 bar (4 fingers)		245
Lion Bar		1 bar		141
M & Ms		1 packet		225
M & Ms, peanut		1 packet		230
Maltesers		1 packet		191
Mars bar		1 std bar		295
Milky Way		1 bar		130
Minstrels		1 packet		244
Revels		1 packet		176
Ripple		1 bar		171
Rolo		1 tube		265
Smarties		1 tube		175
Snickers		1 bar		315
Toffee Crisp		1 bar		245
Topic		1 bar		248
Treets		1 packet		235
Twix		1 bar		263
Yorkie, almond		1 bar		325
Yorkie, milk		1 bar		345
Yorkie, raisin & biscuit		1 bar		285

Branded Sweets

Asda

assorted ecclairs	463			
cola bottles	358			
dairy fudge	434			
fruit pastilles	319			
hard gums	342			
jelly babies	334			

Food Category or Brand	Calories /100g	Portion	Size /g	Calories /port
sherbet fruit	402			
toffee	448			
wine gums	335			
Barker & Dobson				
assorted toffees	393			
barley sugar	321			
buttered selection	393			
chewy mints	500			
chocolate dragées	464			
chocolate peanuts	553			
chocolate raisins	375			
cream or Devon toffee	428			
Everton mints	375			
fruit-flavoured drops	321			
fruit-flavoured jellies	303			
fruit-flavoured pastilles	250			
glacé mints	321			
liquorice caramel	428			
menthol & eucalyptus	500			
mint imperials	393			
nut brittle	428			
old English toffee	428			
sherbet bon-bons	500			
toasted coconut marshmallows	393			
treacle toffee	428			
wine gums	178			
Bassett				
American hard gums	332			
cream rock	357			
jelly babies	325			
jelly beans	339			
liquorice allsorts	357			
mint imperials	378			

Food Category or Brand	Calories /100g	Portion	Size /g	Calories /port
real fruit gums	296			
real fruit pastilles	307			
wine gums	314			

Callard & Bowser Nuttall
barley sugar		1 sweet		25
boiled sweet		1 sweet		20
Brazil nut toffee		1 sweet		40
butterscotch		1 sweet		25
dessert nougat		1 sweet		55
extra strong mint		1 sweet		5
Mintoes		1 sweet		15
treacle toffee		1 sweet		40

Dextrosol
dextro energy tablets		1 sweet		10

Fox's
Glacier fruit or mint		1 packet		140

Fryers
Hacks	357			
Victory V gums	303			
Victory V lozenges	339			

Mars
Lockets		1 packet		155
Skittles		1 packet		175
Starburst		1 packet		175
Tunes		1 packet		135

Paynes
peanut & raisin Poppets		1 packet		210
raisin Poppets		1 packet		180

Food Category or Brand	Calories /100g	Portion	Size /g	Calories /port
Sharps				
bon-bons, all flavours		1 sweet		25
Brazil nuts		1 sweet		30
chocolate eclair		1 sweet		45
chocolate mint cream		1 sweet		40
real fruit jelly		1 sweet		30
St Michael (Marks & Spencer)				
buttermints	428			
chocolate eclairs	482			
chocolate raisins	414			
Devon toffees	460			
fruit gums	327			
fruit pastilles	334			
mint humbugs	407			
Terry's				
sugared almonds	464			
truffle selection	486			
Trebor				
aniseed imperials		1 sweet		20
bon-bons, all flavours		1 sweet		25
chocolate fudge		1 sweet		45
dairy fudge		1 sweet		45
jelly babies		1 sweet		20
jelly beans		1 sweet		10
mint cream fondants		1 sweet		30
raisin fudge		1 sweet		40
Turkish Delight		1 sweet		25
Trident				
sugarless chewing gum		1 stick		5

Food Category or Brand	Calories /100g	Portion	Size /g	Calories /port
Waitrose				
assorted toffees	453			
chocolate eclairs	465			
dolly mixture	396			
fruit pastilles	340			
jelly babies	293			
mint humbugs	415			
wine gums	332			
Wrigley's				
Doublemint		1 stick		10
Hubba Bubba, all flavours		1 stick		15
Orbit, all flavours		1 stick		10
PK, all flavours		1 pellet		5
Branded Cereal Bars				
Boots Shapers				
caramel	352	1 bar	25	90
chocolate & orange	374	1 bar	25	94
cranberry & apple	391	1 bar	25	98
crispy caramel	400	1 bar	24	95
mint	378	1 bar	25	98
strawberry	374	1 bar	22	81
Turkish Delight	310	1 bar	32	98
Cluster				
apple & hazelnut	381			
apricot & chocolate chip	384			
hazelnut & raisin	418			
peanut & almond	463			
Holly Mills				
apple & cardamom	424	1 bar		170
apple & hazelnut	490	1 bar		147
apricot honey	277	1 bar		83

Food Category or Brand	Calories /100g	Portion	Size /g	Calories /port
apricot malt	263	1 bar		79
banana fruit	345	1 bar		93
banana munch	475	1 bar		142
carob chip	490	1 bar		147
crunchy slice	492	1 bar		187
fibre-time snack	387	1 bar		147
oat, apple & raisin	441	1 bar		165
oat, apricot & almond	461	1 bar		203
oat & sesame seed	453	1 bar		135
oat & sunflower seed	455	1 bar		136
protein	416	1 bar		183
roasted peanut	520	1 bar		155
SQUARE SNACKS				
crunchy oat & nut	407	1 bar		187
muesli	432	1 bar		216
oat, fruit & nut	414	1 bar		174

Kalibu

	Calories /100g	Portion	Size /g	Calories /port
carob chips	493	1 bar		139
carob-coated peanuts	510	1 bar		144
carob-coated peanuts & raisins	465	1 bar		131
carob-coated raisins	431	1 bar		122
crunchy bran & raisin	432	1 bar		122
fruit & nut (no sugar)	483	1 bar		136
fruit & nut (raw sugar)	463	1 bar		131
orange (no sugar)	493	1 bar		139
orange (raw sugar)	493	1 bar		139
peanut butters	646	1 bar		182
peanut (no sugar)	507	1 bar		143
peppermint (no sugar)	493	1 bar		139
plain (no sugar)	493	1 bar		139
plain (raw sugar)	493	1 bar		139
raspberry yoghurt	411			

Food Category or Brand	Calories /100g	Portion	Size /g	Calories /port
yoghurt break	526			
yoghurt-coated peanuts	546			
yoghurt-coated peanuts & raisins	508			
yoghurt-coated raisins	442			
SNACK BARS				
banana chew	326	1 bar		92
cherry chew	409	1 bar		115
fruit bar	338	1 bar		95
ginger fudge	414	1 bar		117
marzipan	435	1 bar		123
raisin	339	1 bar		96
Jordan's Original Crunchy Bars				
apple & bran	394	1 bar		131
coconut & honey	416	1 bar		139
honey & almonds	412	1 bar		137
orange & carob	420	1 bar		140
Mars Tracker Bars				
chocolate chip, large		1 bar		180
chocolate chip, small		1 bar		130
roasted nut, large		1 bar		185
roasted nut, small		1 bar		135
Quaker				
chocolate chip, chewy		1 bar		110
fruit & new, chewy		1 bar		110
harvest apple & raisin, chewy		1 bar		105
mint chocolate chip, chewy		1 bar		110
peanut crunch		1 bar		85
raisin crunch		1 bar		80

Food Category or Brand	Calories /100g	Portion	Size /g	Calories /port
Sainsbury's				
choc chip & nut		per bar		119
raisin & hazelnut		per bar		120
Weetabix				
Alpen natural crunch		1 bar		115
apple & hazelnut		1 bar		110
apricot & chocolate chip		1 bar		110
chocolate chip & raisin		1 bar		110
orange & chocolate chip		1 bar		115

Vegetables, Pulses and Prepared Salads

Vegetables

Fresh vegetables are low in energy content; between 70 and 90 per cent of their weight is water, the small amount of carbohydrate they contain is principally starch and, with few exceptions, they are fat-free. Their nutritional benefit comes from the fact that they are great sources of vitamins, minerals and fibre.

The commonly-eaten vegetable with the highest starch is the potato: boiled potatoes are 17 per cent carbohydrate; roast potatoes 26 per cent carbohydrate and 4 or 5 per cent fat. Potatoes mashed with butter and milk will be about 15 per cent carbohydrate and 5 per cent fat.

Home-made chips (French fries) are 30 to 35 per cent carbohydrate and the fat content can be anywhere from 7 to 12 per cent; commercial frozen French fries often end up with a lower water content than home-made and as a result the carbohydrate can exceed 40 per cent and the fat can be over 20 per cent. Baked oven chips usually end up at 30 per cent carbohydrate and only 4 per cent fat. In general terms thin-cut and crinkle-cut chips have a higher fat content because a greater proportion of the potato is available to be fried.

Among the more exotic vegetables, cassava and plantain are also high in starch. Plantain in particular, as it is often cooked with butter, becomes a very high-calorie dish.

Pulses

Pulses are the dried seeds of the leguminosa family of plants – that is, peas and beans. They all have a very high protein content, but for the most part this protein is the non-essential or plant-type as opposed to the essential, animal-type. The exception is the soya bean.

Pulses are a good source of B vitamins, minerals and fibre. Fresh pulses are also rich in vitamin C, but this vitamin is lost in the drying process.

Beans and pulses of all kinds are high in starch; some of the calorific values given for these are for the dried bean: dried chick peas, black-eyed peas and the like contain about 10 per cent water – after cooking the water content is between 65 and 70 per cent. In a fresh bean the water content may be over 90 per cent.

Salads

The salads covered here are the commercially-prepared kind bought in supermarkets. The fattening element usually comes from the added mayonnaise or other sauce. If you make up your own, refer to 'Vegetables' below and the section on **Fats and Oils**.

Food Category or Brand	Calories /100g	Portion /g	Size /port	Calories
Generic Vegetables				
Ackee				
raw	154	1 serving	100	154

Food Category or Brand	Calories /100g	Portion /g	Size /port	Calories
Agar				
canned	5	1 serving	100	5
Alfalfa Sprouts				
fresh	7	1 serving	100	7
Artichokes				
globe, boiled	7	1 head		5
Jerusalem, boiled	20	1 serving		20
Asparagus				
boiled	9	6 stalks	100	9
Aubergine				
raw	15			
Avocado				
raw (without stone)	93	whole	85	79
Bamboo Shoots				
canned	18	1 serving	85	15
Beansprouts				
canned	9	1 serving	85	7
fresh, raw	35	1 serving	85	28
Bean Threads				
dried	393	1 serving	85	334
Beetroot				
boiled	44	1 serving	80	35
raw	28			
Breadfruit				
raw	107	1 serving	85	91

Food Category or Brand	Calories /100g	Portion /g	Size /port	Calories
Broccoli				
tops, boiled	14	1 serving	100	14
Brussels Sprouts				
boiled	16	1 serving	100	16
raw	32			
Cabbage				
red, raw	20	1 serving	85	15
savoy, boiled	9	1 serving	85	5
savoy, raw	26	1 serving	85	20
spring, boiled	8	1 serving	85	5
winter, boiled	8	1 serving	85	5
winter, raw	25	1 serving	85	20
Carrot				
canned	19	1 serving	85	16
old, boiled	19	1 serving	85	15
old, raw	23	1 serving	85	20
young, boiled	21	1 serving	85	15
Cassava				
fresh	154	1 serving	85	131
Cauliflower				
boiled	11	1 serving	85	10
raw	25	1 serving	85	21
Celeriac				
boiled	14	1 serving	85	10
Celery				
boiled	5	1 serving	85	4
raw	9	1 serving	85	5

Food Category or Brand	Calories /100g	Portion /g	Size /port	Calories
Chicory				
raw	9			
Chinese Leaves				
boiled	18	1 serving	120	22
raw	11	1 serving	120	12
Chinese Waterchestnuts				
canned	50			
Chillies				
fresh, flesh only	21			
hot, no seeds	65			
hot, dried	338			
Chives				
raw	36	1 serving	85	33
Courgettes				
raw	18	1 serving	120	22
Cucumber				
raw	9	½ cucumber	100	9
Eggplant				
see Aubergine				
Endive				
raw	11			
Fennel				
boiled	11	1 serving	85	10
raw	11	1 serving	85	10

Food Category or Brand	Calories /100g	Portion /g	Size /port	Calories
Horseradish				
raw	60			
Kale				
without stems, cooked	25	1 serving	120	28
without stems, raw	32	1 serving	120	35
Leeks				
boiled	25	1 serving	125	30
raw	30			
Lettuce				
raw	11	whole	200	20
Mangetout				
boiled	43	1 serving	120	48
raw	57	1 serving	120	63
Marrow				
boiled	7	1 serving	125	10
Mint				
fresh	11	1 serving	100	
Mushrooms				
fried	217	1 serving	85	185
raw	7	1 serving	125	10
Mustard & Cress				
raw	10	1 serving	100	10
Okra				
raw	18	1 serving	120	21

Food Category or Brand	Calories /100g	Portion /g	Size /port	Calories
Onions				
boiled	13	1 serving	85	10
fried	355	1 serving	100	355
raw	23			
spring, raw	36	6 onions	50	20
Parsley				
raw	21			
Parsnips				
boiled	56	1 serving	125	70
raw	49			
Peppers				
sweet, boiled	18	1 serving	85	15
sweet, raw	20	1 serving	85	18
Pimento				
canned	21	1 serving	100	21
Plantain				
green, boiled	125	1 serving	120	150
green, raw	114	1 serving	120	137
ripe, fried in butter	268	1 serving	120	351
Potatoes				
baked in skin (flesh only)	104	1 potato	100	105
baked in skin (with skin)	84	1 potato	150	125
boiled	80	1 potato	120	100
chips	239	1 serving	120	285
mashed (margarine & milk)	120	1 serving	150	180
new, boiled	75	1 serving	120	90
roast	123	1 serving	120	145

Food Category or Brand	Calories /100g	Portion /g	Size /port	Calories
Pumpkin				
canned	33	pie filling	85	30
raw	15			
Radishes				
raw	15	3 radishes	45	10
Salsify				
boiled	18	1 serving	100	18
Seakale				
boiled	8	1 serving	100	8
Spinach				
boiled	26	1 serving	100	26
Spring Greens				
boiled	10	1 serving	100	10
Spring Onions				
raw	36	1 serving	100	36
Squash				
cooked, baked	67	1 serving	150	100
raw	36			
Swedes				
boiled	18	1 serving	120	20
raw	21			
Sweetcorn				
cob		whole		155
frozen	89	1 serving	120	107

Food Category or Brand	Calories /100g	Portion /g	Size /port	Calories
Sweet Potatoes				
boiled	80	1 serving	120	95
Tomatillos				
raw	32	1 serving	120	38
Tomatoes				
fried	71	1 serving	10	7
raw	14	1 large tomato	150	20
sun-dried		1 tomato		5
Turnips				
boiled	11	1 serving	120	15
raw	18			
tops, boiled	11	1 serving	10	1
Wakame				
raw	45	1 serving	120	50
Watercress				
raw	15	1 serving	50	10
Yams				
boiled	114	1 serving	120	137
Zucchini				
see Courgettes				

Generic Pulses
Aduki Beans

boiled	125			
dried	275			

Food Category or Brand	Calories /100g	Portion Size /g	Calories /port
Baked Beans			
canned	93		
Black-eyed Peas			
dried	314		
boiled	118		
Borlotti Beans			
canned	168		
Butter Beans			
boiled	103		
dried	293		
Chick Peas			
boiled	150		
raw	325		
Flageolet			
boiled	114		
canned	114		
dried	350		
French Beans			
boiled	7		
Garbanzo Beans			
see Chick Peas			
Haricot Beans			
boiled	95		
dried	289		

Food Category or Brand	Calories /100g	Portion	Size /g	Calories /port
Kidney Beans				
boiled	103			
canned	100			
dried	268			
Mung Beans				
boiled	93			
dried	282			
Peas				
canned	86			
dried, boiled	100			
dried, raw	275			
fresh, boiled	49			
fresh, raw	64			
frozen or dried	64			
split, dried, boiled	116			
split, dried, raw	303			
Pinto Beans				
boiled	139			
dried	332			
Runner Beans				
raw	15			
Soya Beans				
boiled	143			
dried	375			

Branded Prepared Salads
Boots Shapers

honey mustard chicken pasta	126	pack		304
Mediterranean tuna pasta salad	97	pack		232

Food Category or Brand	Calories /100g	Portion	Size /g	Calories /port
mushroom & pesto pasta salad	146	pack		313
prawn cocktail pasta salad	82	pack		250
tomato & mozzarella salad	114	pack		216

Safeway

carrot & nut salad	173			
celery, nut & sultana salad	177			
coleslaw salad	146			
Italian style pasta salad	150			
pasta with sweetcorn & tuna salad	178			
pesto pasta salad	144			
potato salad	223			
prawn & pasta salad	141			
tuna niçoise salad	186			
vegetable salad	219			
Waldorf salad	300			

Sainsbury's

3 bean salad	161	pot		405
economy coleslaw	108	pot		486
Florida salad	158	pot		396
guacamole		pot		212
hummus		pot		532
reduced calorie coleslaw	101	pot		252
reduced calorie potato salad	103	pot		261
Waldorf salad	233	pot		582

St Michael (Marks & Spencer)

beetroot salad	44			
California style salad	24			
cheese layer	205			
coleslaw	180			
crispy salad mixed	35			

Food Category or Brand	Calories /100g	Portion	Size /g	Calories /port
Greek salad	178			
green salad	15			
Italian rice salad	125			
new potato salad	91			
prawn layer	75			
tomato & basil	96			
wild roquelle	31			
Tesco				
brown rice	164	1 pot	250	410
brown rice & vegetables	106	1 pot	250	265
carrot & nut	176	1 pot	250	440
celery, nut & sultana	216	1 pot	250	540
three-bean	144	1 pot	250	360
vegetable	183	1 pot	227	415
Waldorf	165	1 pot	200	330
FRESH				
continental	15	1 packet	200	30
continental mixed	17	1 packet	200	35
country	27	1 packet	200	55
crunchy cauliflower	57	1 packet	200	115
crunchy nut	55	1 packet	200	110
four seasons	17	1 packet	200	35
high-fibre	65	1 packet	200	130
summer	17	1 packet	200	35
Waitrose				
bean with chilli	124			
beansprout	29			
cabbage & walnut	90			
carrot & poppy seed	114			
carrot with sultanas	68			
cherry tomato	17			
Chinese leaf/sweetcorn	43			

Food Category or Brand	Calories /100g	Portion	Size /g	Calories /port
fresh spinach	19			
Indonesian	40			
mixed	29			
mushroom rice	178			
pesto pasta	109			
potato & bacon	202			
potato & spring onion	132			
spicy pasta	115			
tuna	239			
Waldorf	70			

Vegetarian Dishes

The dishes included here are manufactured ready-made meals aimed at the 'vegetarian' market. You will also find some vegetarian items in the **Ready-made Meals** section. Some of these dishes would not be suitable for vegans as they contain cow's milk, eggs, etc.

This section includes vegetable-based meat substitutes, such as TVP (textured vegetable protein) and Quorn, which is a myco-protein grown from a tiny fungus. Quorn is low in fat and saturated fat, cholesterol-free and a good source of fibre. A typical serving of Quorn contains 55 calories as against the 300 calories in a portion of roast chicken which included some skin. A portion of soya mince (TVP) is about 80 calories.

Tofu is soya bean curd: the firm type has been pressed and is useful for deep-frying; the most common version is called silken tofu and has the consistency of cream – it is usually made into dips and sauces. Tofu is low in calories and fats.

Vegetarian dishes are often thought of as 'healthy' but that does not always mean 'slimming'. The features to watch for are the sauces and binders used in these recipes. Manufacturers may use fattening binders to hold their 'roasts' and 'burgers' together. Cheese-based sauces (as in cauliflower cheese) are very fattening.

Food Category or Brand	Calories /100g	Portion	Size /g	Calories /port
Branded Vegetarian Meals				
Asda				
cauliflower cheese	117	1 packet	227	265
macaroni cheese	157	1 packet	300	470
spinach & ricotta canneloni	121	1 packet	300	363
tomato & cheese pasta bake	109	1 packet	550	599
vegetable lasagne	108	1 packet	300	324
vegetable tikka masala	107	1 packet	340	362
vegetable spring rolls	184	each	93	171
Batchelors Beanfeasts				
American style		1 packet		345
Chinese style		1 packet		240
Birds Eye Wall's				
cauliflower cheese		meal		312
cheese & broccoli bake		1/2 pack		400
cheese, onion & tomato lasagne		meal		375
crispy vegetable finger		each		30
macaroni cheese		meal		285
original vegetable quarterpounder		each		114
roasted vegetable & tomato pasta		meal		350
vegetable Tuscany bake		1/2 pack		400
Cauldron Foods				
carrot & coriander pâté	143			
chickpea & black olive pâté	166			
chilli flavour tofu burger	214			

Food Category or Brand	Calories /100g	Portion	Size /g	Calories /port
marinated tofu	102			
original tofu	90			
smoked tofu	116			
spicy bean burger	276			
tomato, lentil & basil pâté	137			
vegetable burgers	164			
vegetable terrine	169			

Dale Pak

GRILLED

cauliflower cheese grill	250	each	100	250
cheese & onion crispbake	257	each	113	290
cheese & vegetable burger	294	each	85	250
crumbled vegetable grill	255	each	100	255
golden vegetable crunchie		each		50
macaroni cheese grill	315	each	100	315
quorn & vegetable crispbake	224	each	85	190
ratatouille grill	240	each	100	240
vegetable burger	199	each	78	155
vegetable grill	182	each	85	155
vegetable grill, curry	182	each	85	155
vegetable salad grill	265	each	100	265
vegetable waffle	192	each	65	125

Findus

broccoli, cheese sauce		1 packet	225	300
cauliflower, cheese sauce		1 packet	225	290
French mushroom flan	224			
French onion flan	231			
green bean & mushroom bake		1 packet	225	270
zucchini lasagne	82			

Food Category or Brand	Calories /100g	Portion	Size /g	Calories /port
Hera				
chilli	310	1 packet	200	620
vegetable bolognese	305	1 packet	200	610
vegetable casserole	310	1 packet	200	620
vegetable cottage pie	349	1 packet	215	750
vegetable curry	313	1 packet	200	625
vegetable goulash	313	1 packet	200	625
vegetable stew, with dumplings	323	1 packet	200	645
vegetable stroganoff	380	1 packet	200	760
vegetable supreme	389	1 packet	149	580
Holland & Barrett				
mild vegetable curry	84	1 can	425	355
mixed bean salad	67	1 can	425	285
onion bhaji		each		230
vegetable spring roll		each		310
vindaloo hot vegetable curry	84	1 can	425	355
Iceland				
cauliflower cheese		1 packet		355
cheese & onion crisp		each		230
vegetable burger		each		165
vegetable grills		each		160
vegetable & nut cutlet		each		165
vegetable sausage		each		130
vegetables au gratin		1 packet		285
vegetable waffles		each		110
Kraft				
cheese & onion pasties	306	each		306
Linda McCartney				
beefless burger	207	each		124
deep country pie	252	each		446

Food Category or Brand	Calories /100g	Portion	Size /g	Calories /port
lasagne	110	each		352
sausage rolls	300	each		195
sausages	212	each		74
southern fried grills	234	each		265

Safeway

cauliflower, broccoli & gruyère	151			
cauliflower cheese	89			
nut cutlets	260			
vegetable chilli	46			
vegetable curry with rice	98			
vegetable cutlets	205			
vegetable pasta bake	65			
vegetable samosa	193			
vegetable spring roll	204			

Sainsbury's

cheese & onion quiche		½ flan		496
potato, cheese and onion pasty		each		228
quorn bolognaise		pack		152
quorn quarter pounder		each		164
quorn sausages		each		57
vegetable lasagne		pack		360
vegetable pie with mushrooms		each		416
vegetarian cottage pie		pack		227
vegetarian moussaka		pack		339

Sharwood's

channa dahl	140	1 can	425	595
chick pea dahl	139	1 can	425	590
mild vegetable curry	65	1 can	405	265
onion bhaji mix	331	1 packet	80	265
potato & pea curry	106	1 can	415	440

Food Category or Brand	Calories /100g	Portion	Size /g	Calories /port
St Michael (Marks & Spencer)				
cheese/cherry tomato bake	160			
feta cheese ravioli	195			
four cheese ravioli	120			
onion/gruyere risotto	175			
pasta & vegetable bake	110			
vegetable & bean hot pot	75			
vegetable tempura spring roll	200			
vegetable/goats cheese tart	230			
vegetable/mozzarella pasta	140			
Waitrose				
leek & stilton quiche	258			
spinach & asparagus forno	131			
spring rolls	274			
vegetable biryani	125			
vegetable curry	58			
vegetable pies	261			

Weight Watchers from Heinz

quorn sweet & sour with rice	286			